Total Parenteral Nutrition

For Churchill Livingstone

Senior Commissioning Editor: Alex Mathieson/Brenda Clark
Project Manager: Jane Shanks
Copyeditor: Anne Trevillion

Total Parenteral Nutrition
A Practical Guide for Nurses

Edited by

Helen Hamilton

Clinical Director, TPN and Line Insertion Service
Department of Parenteral Nutrition
Oxford Radcliffe NHS Trust
Oxford, UK

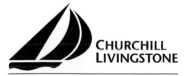

CHURCHILL
LIVINGSTONE

EDINBURGH LONDON NEW YORK PHILADELPHIA ST LOUIS SYDNEY TORONTO 2000

CHURCHILL LIVINGSTONE
An imprint of Harcourt Publishers Limited

© Harcourt Publishers Limited 2000

🕮 is a registered trademark of Harcourt Publishers Limited

The right of Helen Hamilton to be identified as editor of this work has
been asserted by her in accordance with the Copyright, Designs and
Patents Act 1988

First published 2000

0 443 06005 3

British Library Cataloguing in Publication Data
A catalogue record for this book is available from the British Library

Library of Congress Cataloging in Publication Data
A catalog record for this book is available from the Library of Congress

Note
Medical knowledge is constantly changing. As new information becomes
available, changes in treatment, procedures, equipment and the use of
drugs become necessary. The editor and the publishers have, as far as it is
possible, taken care to ensure that the information given in this text is
accurate and up to date. However, readers are strongly advised to
confirm that the information, especially with regard to drug usage,
complies with the latest legislation and standards of practice.

The
publisher's
policy is to use
**paper manufactured
from sustainable forests**

Printed in China

Contents

Contributors **vii**

Preface **ix**

1. What is parenteral nutrition? **1**
   Christopher Pennington

2. The multidisciplinary team **17**
   Jill Hudson

3. Patient assessment **31**
   Clare Burnett

4. Choosing the appropriate catheter for patients requiring parenteral nutrition **55**
   Helen Hamilton

5. Preparing the patient for central venous catheter insertion **83**
   Helen Balsdon

6. The insertion of a central venous catheter for parenteral nutrition **101**
   Helen Hamilton

7. Nursing management **137**
   Jan Tait

8. Dietetic aspects of parenteral nutrition **173**
   Helen Dewar

9. Complications **187**
   Louise Sherliker

10. Home parenteral nutrition **205**
    Sally Magnay

11. Living with parenteral nutrition: a patient's perspective **219**
    Stephen McManus

12. Conclusion **227**
    Katherine Fermo

Index **235**

Contributors

Helen L Balsdon BSc (Hons) Cancer Care
Staff Nurse, Haematology and Bone Marrow Transplant Unit, Oxford
Radcliffe NHS Trust, Oxford, UK

Clare A Burnett BA (Hons) Nursing Studies BA Children's Nursing
Paediatric Gastroenterology Nurse Specialist, Oxford Radcliffe NHS
Trust, Oxford, UK

Helen Dewar BSc (Hons) Nutrition SRD DipADP
Senior Dietitian, Oxford Radcliffe NHS Trust, Oxford, UK

Katherine Fermo BA (Hons)
Completing Master's in Public Health, Victorian Consortium for Public
Health, Melbourne, Australia; formerly Clinical Nurse Specialist, TPN
and Line Insertion Service, Oxford Radcliffe NHS Trust, Oxford, UK

Helen Hamilton RGN
Clinical Director, TPN and Line Insertion Team, Oxford Radcliffe NHS
Trust, Oxford, UK

Jill Hudson RGN BA (Hons)
Clinical Nurse Specialist, TPN and Line Insertion Team, Oxford Radcliffe
NHS Trust, Oxford, UK

Michael Kettlewell MA MChir FRCS
Consultant Surgeon and Medical Director, Oxford Radcliffe NHS Trust,
Oxford, UK

Steven McManus BA (Hons)
Health Care Studies, Post Grad Cert. Evidence-Based Health Care
Clinical Nurse Specialist, TPN and Line Insertion Team, Oxford Radcliffe
NHS Trust, Oxford, UK

Sally Magnay RGN
Clinical Nurse Specialist, TPN and Line Insertion Team, Oxford Radcliffe
NHS Trust, Oxford, UK

Christopher R Pennington BSc MD FRCP FRCPE
Professor, Consultant Physician in Gastroenterology, Tayside University
Hospitals NHS Trust, Dundee, UK

Louise Sherliker RGN DipHSM MSc
Ward Manager, Haematology and Bone Marrow Transplant Unit, Oxford
Radcliffe NHS Trust, Oxford, UK

Jan Tait RGN RM
Nurse Practitioner in Gastroenterology, Tayside University Hospitals
NHS Trust, Dundee, UK

Preface

Parenteral nutrition has come of age. It has been part of the clinical remit for thirty years, but is still often misunderstood and inappropriately used. Nearly thirty years ago Hill and Bistrain demonstrated that malnutrition was common in the hospitals of affluent countries and was not the preserve of the chronically starved developing world. Furthermore, these workers found that malnutrition in hospital was more common the longer patients were in hospital and was also more likely following surgery associated with post-operative complications.

For many years parenteral nutrition was seen as a sophisticated and complex modern therapy bedevilled by complications. However, time has shown that nutrition can be given safely and successfully to patients whose intestines are either temporarily or permanently out of commission. Success, however, only comes with scrupulous attention to detail. This book aims to assist nurses and junior doctors to consider the necessary elements regarding the assessment, selection, implementation and monitoring of patients receiving intravenous nutrition.

Effective nutritional support of severely ill patients has always been a team matter with nurses, doctors, pharmacists and dietitians all playing important parts in restoring these patients to good health. Recently we have shown that the insertion of the central feeding lines and the delivery of the service can be effectively and efficiently nurse led.

This book is written by a series of distinguished authors widely versed in the provision of parenteral nutrition. The book is essentially practical and leads the reader through the main issues surrounding parenteral nutrition, from the insertion of feeding catheters to the committee skills necessary to maintain and develop the service for the ongoing benefit of patients

Oxford
1999

Michael Kettlewell
Helen Hamilton

What is parenteral nutrition?

Christopher Pennington

Introduction
Definitions
Indications
Nutrient solutions
Nutrient delivery

Patient monitoring
Complications
Resources for PN
Home parenteral nutrition

INTRODUCTION

The intestine has two major functions: the digestion and absorption of nutrients, and its action as a barrier against lumenal microorganisms and toxins. Intestinal failure may lead to nutrient deficiency and also to the translocation and permeation of microorganisms and toxins. Patients with this condition have three problems: malnutrition and electrolyte imbalance; infection and possibly multiorgan failure; and symptoms such as diarrhoea and vomiting. They also have the clinical features of the underlying disease.

Before the advent of artificial nutritional support, prolonged intestinal failure led to the death of the patient. The development of intravenous feeding has transformed the outlook for patients undergoing intestinal surgery, those in intensive care, and those with permanent intestinal failure due to inflammatory disease, short bowel syndrome or other intestinal pathology. This form of treatment is required to prevent or treat malnutrition when the intestinal function is not available or is severely impaired. The possibility in the future of using specific nutrients to modify the inflammatory or the immune response and improve intestinal function may add another dimension to nutritional therapy.

Parenteral nutrition, otherwise known as intravenous nutrition, involves the intravenous infusion of nutrients. The required nutrients, electrolytes, trace elements, vitamins and water, in addition to sources of energy and nitrogen, are compounded in a large collapsible bag, typically 3 L in capacity, and infused via an infusion pump through a venous catheter or cannula.

This chapter reviews the practice and role of parenteral nutrition for the benefit of clinicians who are unfamiliar with this treatment; it is an introduction to the methodology that is addressed in more detail in the following chapters.

DEFINITIONS

The various terms used in the literature can be confusing. Definitions have become more precise, rendering some previous terminology obsolete.

Intravenous hyperalimentation (IVH) was the name given to the provision of amino acids and hypertonic dextrose solutions in excess of the patient's requirements. Such excessive nutrient administration was given in a futile attempt to induce a positive nitrogen balance in catabolic patients. This form of feeding is dangerous, wasteful and obsolete.

Total parenteral nutrition (TPN) may be interpreted as referring to the provision of either the total spectrum of nutrients, or all the nutrient needs, exclusively by the intravenous route. *Supplemental parenteral nutrition* (SPN) may refer to the administration of some nutritional substrates or part of the whole spectrum of nutrient needs intravenously. The use of the terms TPN and SPN may lead to confusion. Although total parenteral nutrition (TPN) is the commonly used terminology, parenteral nutrition (PN) is preferred.

Central parenteral nutrition (CPN) and *peripheral parenteral nutrition* (PPN) relate to the use of central or peripheral venous access for nutrient delivery. Confusion may arise in relation to peripherally inserted central catheters (PICC). Consequently, it is suggested that the words 'peripheral' and 'central' are used to describe the primary point of venous access. Thus, access at or below the antecubital fossa is considered to be peripheral; catheters inserted into the superior vena cava or a tributary are described as central, and PICC lines (infrequently used in UK practice) are described as peripherally inserted central catheters (Pennington 1996).

INDICATIONS

Parenteral nutrition is required when the intestine is unavailable or the intestinal function is insufficient to absorb or digest an adequate supply of nutrients on a temporary or a permanent basis. Parenteral nutrition should not be used when it is possible to meet nutritional needs using the oral or enteral routes; enteral feeding is cheaper, safer, and is associated with physiological advantages. However, in many patients PN will be needed to supplement inadequate intestinal absorption, and in some it will be required to meet all nutrient needs when the intestine is not available.

Examples of diseases that may lead to the need for PN are given in Box 1.1. Following intestinal surgery, small intestinal function recovers before gastric motility. The use of nasojejunal feeding or surgically placed jejunostomy, with or without simultaneous gastric aspiration, may avoid or reduce the need for PN in many patients.

The time at which nutritional support should be initiated will depend on individual circumstances. Malnutrition will impair organ function, for

---

Box 1.1 Examples of indications for parenteral nutrition

Short-term parenteral nutrition
- Intestinal surgery
- Severe pancreatitis
- Mucositis

Long-term parenteral nutrition
- Extreme short bowel syndrome
- Radiation enteritis
- Severe Crohn's disease
- Hollow visceral myopathy

---

example muscle strength and stamina, before significant clinically measurable change in structure is detectable. Such impairment has implications for respiratory reserve. Starvation for more than 7 days has been shown to be detrimental in normal individuals, and shorter periods of inadequate intake are probably detrimental in patients with pre-existing malnutrition or in others who are hypercatabolic in association with sepsis, trauma or other metabolic stress. Nutritional support should therefore be started in all individuals exposed to 7 or more days without oral intake, in those anticipated to be at risk of such a duration of restricted intake, or earlier in compromised patients (British Society of Gastroenterology 1997). In patients who are not septic, when the problem is primarily inadequate intestinal function, PN can prevent or reverse nutritional depletion. During the acute phase of illness, for example with trauma, burns and sepsis, inflammatory mediators known as cytokines induce muscle wasting, aggravating the effect of anorexia and intestinal failure. Under these circumstances nutritional support will reduce the rate of tissue wasting, but will not prevent it (Askanazi et al 1980, Hill 1992). Thus early nutritional support is indicated under these circumstances.

Many patients will only require short-term PN; for example, patients in whom the use of the intestine is not anticipated in the early postoperative period after major excisional surgery, those with severe pancreatitis, those with mucositis following chemotherapy, and a minority of patients with inflammatory bowel disease. Parenteral nutrition is often needed in patients with multiorgan failure where nutritional requirements cannot be met by enteral nutrition alone. The duration of PN required in these patients is determined by return of gastrointestinal function and may often be 2 weeks or less (Payne-James et al 1995).

Long-term PN is employed in patients with prolonged episodes of intestinal failure. Examples include severe inflammatory disease such as radiation enteritis and Crohn's disease with extensive resection; motility disorders such as scleroderma and hollow visceral myopathy resulting in pseudo-obstruction; and extreme short bowel syndrome of any aetiology. Some of these patients will need treatment with home PN.

Box 1.2 Examples of trace elements that are important in humans	
Iron	Zinc
Copper	Manganese
Selenium	Chromium
Cobalt	Iodine
Molybdenum	Fluorine

NUTRIENT SOLUTIONS

Patients who require PN should receive as complete a range of nutrients as possible. The nutrient solutions include amino acids, glucose, lipids, electrolytes, vitamins, trace elements and water. Trace elements are nutrients that are required in very small amounts and constitute less than 0.01% of the total body weight. Those elements that are important in the human are listed in Box 1.2.

Energy

The majority of adult patients are maintained in the range of 25–35 non-protein kilocalories per kilogram body weight per day (Elia 1995). Parenteral energy needs are reduced during periods of weaning from PN to enteral nutrition and when PN is used as an adjunct to enteral feeding. Energy should be supplied below the estimated needs when initiating PN in the severely depleted or critically ill patient. An upper limit of 40 kilocalories per kilogram should not be exceeded. The administration of excess glucose is associated with hyperglycaemia and consequent increased respiratory demands that may cause dyspnoea or difficulty in weaning from mechanical ventilation. Most patients receive energy in the form of glucose and lipid solutions that are compounded with the other nutrients in the single bag, with lipid supplying 30–50% of the energy needs. Lipid solutions supply essential fatty acids, and in these solutions the osmolality is lower than in those in which all the non-protein energy needs are met with glucose. This permits the infusion of some solutions into peripheral veins.

Nitrogen

Nitrogen is supplied in the vast majority of patients as a balance of crystalline amino acids. With the provision of adequate energy, nitrogen balance can be obtained in most patients with 0.2 g nitrogen per kg body weight. Although some patients may utilise more nitrogen, exceeding 0.3 g/kg does not confer benefit and may be dangerous.

Water and electrolytes

Standard solutions provide 80 mmol of sodium and 60 mmol of potassium in a volume of 2.0–3.0 L. Patients with high-output jejunostomies and high-output fistulae will need additional water and electrolytes; the amount can be estimated from the measurement of the content and volume of the fistula fluid. Malnourished oedematous patients will need small-volume feeds with reduced sodium content. Sodium and water retention can also be a problem when malnourished patients are provided with regimens in which all the non-protein energy is supplied as carbohydrate, rather than with lipid-containing regimens, owing to the influence of insulin on sodium transport.

The major intracellular electrolytes – potassium, magnesium and phosphorus – are also required. Serum concentrations of these electrolytes may fall rapidly once adequate energy and nitrogen have been provided, owing to the enhanced cellular uptake under the influence of insulin. Serum concentrations should be monitored daily in the early phases of treatment, especially in severely malnourished patients, and sufficient amounts given to maintain serum levels within the normal range.

Magnesium deficiency is particularly common in undernourished alcoholic patients and in patients with excessive gastrointestinal losses, for example Crohn's disease; it may lead to hypokalaemia and hypocalcaemia, resistant to the respective supplements. Hypophosphataemia is relatively common and potentially dangerous; it may present with thrombocytopenia, weakness, confusion or cardiac dysrhythmia, and may lead to death. The administration of glucose leads to insulin secretion, which increases the transport of glucose and phosphate into the cell; this may result in profound hypophosphataemia in the previously malnourished patient (Solomon and Kirby 1990). Patients should receive phosphate replacement before commencing PN.

Where serum concentrations of electrolytes are high, principally in patients with renal failure, a reduction in the electrolyte content of the bag, especially potassium, is required.

Trace elements

Trace element requirements can be met in most patients by the prescription of a commercially available trace element solution. Measurement of trace element status is recommended in the severely depleted patient and the patient who requires long-term treatment.

Vitamins

Vitamin requirements are met with commercially available compounded solutions that are added to the bag shortly before infusion. Specific recommendations from the American Medical Association have increased the suggested provision of water-soluble vitamins above the normal estimated daily requirements. The additional provision is considered necessary to restore tissue depletion, facilitate new tissue synthesis, and cover presumed increased requirements associated with disease (although this is not based on scientific measurement). The degradation of vitamins in the nutrient solution is also important as it reduces substantially the amount of nutrient that is delivered to the patient. Sunlight will degrade some forms of vitamin A with the loss of 40–98% during a 24 h infusion. Protection from sunlight will prevent this problem, and the use of multi-layer bags will greatly reduce the loss of vitamin C, which is susceptible to oxidation.

Novel substrates

The management of stressed patients remains difficult. The provision of PN can retard, but not prevent, tissue wasting. The recognition of the importance of intestinal barrier function and the potential role of conditionally essential amino acids such as glutamine and arginine on intestinal and immune function has attracted much interest. Glutamine is not available in conventional amino acid solutions because of concern about stability. Recently glutamine in the form of a dipeptide has been licensed for use in the critically ill patient. Glutamine is required as a fuel for the enterocyte, which lines the small intestine and is involved in the absorption of nutrients. By improving the intestinal barrier function it is hoped to reduce the translocation of microorganisms, which is thought to promote systemic sepsis and further enhance the inflammatory response.

Provision of the three branched-chain amino acids, leucine, isoleucine and valine, in amounts greater than that supplied in standard nutrient solutions has been suggested for the management of the stressed patient and patients with portal systemic encephalopathy associated with chronic liver disease. At present, branched-chain-enriched amino acid solutions should be limited to those patients with severe liver disease who require PN and in whom portal systemic encephalopathy is associated with conventional solutions and is not controlled by conventional treatment.

The compounding of nutrient solutions

Nutrient solutions are compounded by the pharmacist under sterile conditions in the pharmacy (Barnett & Cosslett 1995). The major pharmaceutical problems are avoidance of infection and ensuring the stability of the lipid emulsion. These can be overcome by including all additives in the pharmacy, and by careful attention to the prescription. For example, the addition of electrolytes has a dramatic effect on the stability of the lipid emulsion – the cations will reduce the surface charge on the droplets, leading to aggregation. The effect that electrolyte ions have on the lipid emulsion is determined by their valency. If there is a requirement for a large quantity of divalent ions such as magnesium or calcium, a separate infusion will be needed. Destabilisation may also follow the addition of heparin for the same reason.

NUTRIENT DELIVERY

All nutrient solutions should be administered through a dedicated feeding line, using a volumetric pump fitted with occlusion and air-in-line alarms, which do not allow free flow. Some authorities recommend the use of in-line filters to remove particulates. These increase the cost of treatment and have not gained widespread acceptance in the UK. The PN solution must be protected from sunlight to prevent degradation of vitamin A.

Cyclical infusion may have physiological and psychological advantages; there is less fluid and fat accumulation, and patients benefit from periods free from infusion (Matuchansky et al 1992). However, continuous infusion is more appropriate for severely stressed patients such as those in the intensive care unit.

The dovetailing of enteral and parenteral feeding is very important. Parenteral nutrition should not stop abruptly. The amount of nutrients infused is reduced as enteral feeding increases. This period of combined enteral feeding and PN is usually short. Decreasing the amount of PN can be achieved by the delivery of a proportion of the volume of solution in the standard bag. This is simpler than compounding a series of individual bags. Most patients can be transferred entirely to enteral or oral feeding when intestinal tolerance of more than half of their total nutrient needs is established.

Wherever possible, some enteral or oral feeding should be encouraged. This may be important in the maintenance of the intestinal architecture and intestinal function and minimises the risks of hepatobiliary complications by stimulating gall bladder contractility. The use of minimal enteral feeding (MEN) in the intensive care patient is recommended.

Parenteral nutrition can be administered by the peripheral or central routes.

Peripheral parenteral nutrition

Peripheral parenteral nutrition is a valuable technique for nutrient delivery that avoids the risk and cost of central catheter insertion, as well as central catheter-related complications (Payne-James & Khawaja 1993). When peripheral veins are available, this route is an option for the management of selected patients in whom the need for parenteral feeding is expected to last for up to 2 weeks. Standard solutions can be used provided they contain lipid, which protects the vein from thrombophlebitis. Peripheral vein feeding will only succeed if meticulous care is taken over catheter management. Where possible, the venous access should be restricted to the administration of nutrient solutions and, if necessary, other veins should be used for the administration of drugs.

Venous access may be obtained through a small cannula (18FG) inserted into a peripheral vein. It is then covered with a sterile adhesive dressing and attached to a short extension set to reduce manipulation of the exit site, and re-sited every 1–2 days. For those patients who are receiving cyclical PN some authorities advocate the removal of the cannula after each infusion. Increasingly, many centres are using fine bore catheters inserted into a vein in the antecubital fossa (22–23FG). There is evidence that polyurethane catheters are less thrombogenic. Although initially more expensive, these catheters may last for prolonged periods. They are ultimately cheaper, more comfortable for the patients, and less demanding on staff time.

The catheters should be managed with appropriate aseptic techniques and the veins inspected for evidence of redness or discomfort at least once a day. Catheters and cannulae should be re-sited if discomfort or redness appears in relation to the catheter or vein.

Pharmaceutical methods have been used for reducing thrombophlebitis, e.g. heparin and hydrocortisone added to the bag or glyceryl trinitrate patches over the vein distal to the insertion site (Tighe et al 1996). The latter may act by venodilatation and increasing blood flow. Studies have demonstrated their efficacy, but the use of these methods can increase the cost of treatment and some authorities consider that they are not necessary.

Central parenteral nutrition

Patients in whom the need for PN is expected to exceed 2 weeks, who lack adequate peripheral veins, or who have unusual needs including fluid restriction and who already have suitable central venous access, are candidates for central venous feeding. The insertion of central venous catheters can lead to potentially serious complications, including damage to surrounding structures and pneumothorax. Caution should be exercised during the placement of catheters in patients with hypoalbuminaemia and hypovolaemia, and in patients with coagulopathies such as liver disease and bone marrow dysfunction. Central venous catheters without a Dacron cuff are often used for medium-term feeding. Patients who need prolonged PN should be equipped with cuffed catheters; however in some cases subcutaneous ports may be preferred. Meticulous catheter care with appropriate protocols is essential to minimise the risk of complications.

PATIENT MONITORING

Patients require careful monitoring of clinical, laboratory and nutritional indices.

Patient assessment before starting PN

Before treatment is commenced the weight and height of the patient should be obtained and temperature, pulse, respiration (TPR) and blood pressure recordings made. Baseline laboratory measurements consist of the following: a full blood count; urea and electrolytes, which should include calcium, magnesium and phosphate; and liver function tests. The need for a micronutrient screen, the measurement of trace elements and vitamins, should be considered in the severely depleted patient and when the need for prolonged treatment is envisaged.

When central lines are used for PN the postinsertion chest X-ray must be viewed to confirm that the catheter is in a satisfactory position and to exclude such immediate complications as pneumothorax.

Clinical monitoring

Where possible patients should be weighed daily, as change in weight is an important guide to fluid balance. The pulse, temperature and blood pressure are monitored as infection may complicate PN, especially with inadequate standards of catheter management. Blood glucose should be measured 12-hourly for the first 2 days. Persistent hyperglycaemia may require supplemental insulin. Blood should also be checked for lipaemia after the first day. It is essential that an accurate fluid balance chart is kept and that fluid losses through vomiting or enterocutaneous fistulae are recorded. Additional intravenous fluids and electrolytes may be needed in a few patients with high-output fistulae. The exit-site dressing should be changed according to local protocol.

Patients who require long-term treatment will also need monitoring with reference to the underlying disease process, and the possibility of transfer from parenteral to enteral feeding following intestinal adaptation should always be considered. Psychological and social aspects should be remembered, especially in patients who receive home PN.

Laboratory monitoring

The frequency with which laboratory measurements are obtained will be governed by the condition of the patient. Unstable patients and patients who are severely malnourished will require more frequent monitoring – usually on a daily basis. In general, urea and electrolytes should be measured every other day, and liver function and haematological tests done twice weekly. Initially, magnesium and phosphate should be included with the electrolyte request; this is especially important in malnourished patients. When patients are severely depleted, or when prolonged treatment is necessary, trace element status is measured at the outset and thereafter every 6–12 weeks.

Serum albumin concentrations increase with nutritional repletion and recovery from illness. The long half-life, in addition to the influence of changes in vascular permeability and fluid balance, limits the value of this measurement as a nutritional marker.

Nutritional monitoring

Nutritional repletion restores function before structure, but at present there are no satisfactory non-invasive bedside tests of function. Some authorities recommend hand grip dynamometry and measurement of respiratory function, although both of these measurements are influenced by other factors. Structural measurements include mid-arm circumference and triceps skinfold thickness when prolonged PN is given.

Continued weight loss over a long period should alert the clinician to the possibility that the PN is inadequate.

COMPLICATIONS

Complications may be considered in three groups: nutritional and metabolic, catheter-related, and the effect of PN on other organ systems (Pennington 1991). Complications can be minimised by the use of appropriate management protocols, and the literature clearly indicates that the best results are achieved in centres where there is an active Nutritional Support Team (Burnham 1995). Some of the important complications are listed in Box 1.3.

Box 1.3 Some complications of PN

Nutritional and metabolic
• Hyperglycaemia
• Hypophosphataemia

Catheter-related
• Infection
• Occlusion
• Central vein thrombosis

Effect on other organ systems
• Hepatic disease
• Biliary track disease
• Bone disease

Nutritional and metabolic complications

Fluid overload, hyperglycaemia and electrolyte imbalance are common potential problems, especially in unstable patients. Patients who are severely malnourished may suffer from the refeeding syndrome. The switch of energy source from endogenous ketones to exogenous glucose will increase insulin secretion, which stimulates the rapid uptake of phosphate, potassium and magnesium into the cell (Solomon & Kirby 1990). Hypophosphataemia, which leads to tissue hypoxia, cardiac dysrhythmia, thrombocytopenia and confusion, can be fatal. Thiamin deficiency precipitated by glucose infusion represents another example of this problem. Careful monitoring is required and additional electrolytes may need to be given to some patients; this particularly applies to phosphate and magnesium. Severely malnourished patients may benefit from initial hypocaloric feeding in which only a proportion of the energy needs are met. Stressed patients are prone to hyperglycaemia, so some of the energy should be provided as lipid. Rebound hypoglycaemia can occur after discontinuing the infusion of concentrated glucose solutions until endogenous insulin levels fall. Tapering the rate of infusion before disconnection can prevent this problem.

Long-term patients who take little nutrition from other sources are at risk of micronutrient deficiencies. Whereas the profile of commercially available trace element solutions has been changed to cover previous deficiencies such as selenium, it is worth remembering that amounts delivered in each nutrition bag are designed to meet estimated daily needs; patients with initial depletion or who do not require a nutrition bag every day (this applies to many of the patients who receive PN at home) are at risk of deficiency, and monitoring is important (Malone et al 1989).

The overprovision of macronutrients such as glucose and amino acids is harmful. Excess glucose will lead to hepatic steatosis and is accompanied by increased respiratory demands and stimulation of the sympathetic nervous system. Amino acid overprovision has been associated with cholestasis in paediatric practice, and the possible alteration in bone metabolism.

Catheter-related complications

Apart from the complications associated with insertion there are four important catheter-related complications: infection, thrombosis, occlusion and fracture.

Catheter-related infection

Three types of infection can be recognised: exit-site infection, tunnel infection and catheter-related septicaemia (CRS).

Exit-site infections usually respond to local dressing complemented by systemic antibiotic therapy. However, clearance will not be successful if the Dacron cuff lies adjacent to the exit site and becomes contaminated. Infection of the tunnel, which can complicate exit-site infection, is characterised by pain and redness; it does not respond to treatment and is an indication for catheter removal. Rarely, tunnel infections may arise from retrograde spread of infection from an infected central vein. This is a very serious problem that reflects previous inadequately treated catheter-related sepsis.

Catheter-related septicaemia is the most serious infection – it can be fatal. In the short term microorganisms may gain access from the exit-site, but after 2 weeks the hub is the most common site of contamination (Linares et al 1985). The problem is usually heralded by pyrexia and rigors during infusion. Diagnosis can be difficult, especially in patients with other sources of sepsis; there may also be other reasons for pyrexia, including venous thrombosis. When this complication is suspected, catheter removal is the safest course of action. However, if venous access is difficult and the need for continuing CPN is anticipated, drawback and peripheral blood cultures should be obtained. Semiquantitative cultures have been used to implicate the line as the primary source of infection, but the use of an endoluminal brush to sample material from the inner wall of the catheter promises more precise and reliable information. While awaiting the results of culture, the central catheter should be locked and the patient given systemic antimicrobial cover against the most likely infecting organisms. Catheter salvage is possible using antibiotic and urokinase locks. Salvage should not be attempted when *Candida* and *Staphylococcus aureus* infections are identified, and it is unlikely to succeed with subcutaneous ports. The potential risk of recrudescent or metastatic infection, including endocarditis and osteomyelitis, should be considered.

The emphasis must be on prevention. The development of catheter care protocols and management by Nutrition Support Teams has almost eliminated the problem.

Central vein thrombosis

Central vein thrombosis tends to develop after treatment for a few weeks. It may be heralded by pyrexia, pulmonary embolism, subclavian vein thrombosis, or occlusion of the superior vena cava with facial swelling. This is a serious problem which impairs venous access and can prove fatal (Pennington 1995).

The diagnosis should be confirmed by bilateral upper limb venography. Rarely in adult practice does the thrombus involve the heart; however, if any new cardiac murmur is heard, transoesophageal echocardiography is recommended.

Thrombosis accompanies the use of concentrated glucose regimens and a proximal location of the catheter tip in the superior vena cava; thrombotic tendency is reduced by compounded lipid-containing emulsions. Early treatment with thrombolytic drugs such as streptokinase is usually effective in restoring venous patency. The use of heparin alone does not lead to significant recanalisation in the short term.

Many authorities use heparin in the nutrient solution as a prophylactic measure. Evidence suggests that there is a need for at least 3 units of heparin per ml of feed solution, although the possible effect on the stability of the emulsion must be considered. There is insufficient evidence to support the routine use of heparin in all patients. Low-dose warfarin may be an effective alternative, notwithstanding interactions between warfarin and the vitamin K derivatives that occur in the lipid emulsions. The need for prophylaxis will depend on individual circumstances. For example, prophylaxis will be required in patients with a thrombotic disorder such as antithrombin 3 deficiency, and in patients who have already developed venous thrombosis. Conversely, anticoagulation is unwise in some patients with active inflammatory disease in whom there is a significant risk of bleeding.

Catheter occlusion

Catheter occlusion may be due to kinking or luminal deposition of fibrin, lipid sludge, or amorphous debris. This is a particular problem with lipid mixes, the tendency to which may be reduced by the use of an ethanol flush (Johnston et al 1992). Ethanol locks of 70% ethanol solution can free catheters that have become partially occluded following the infusion of a lipid mix. When there is evidence for fibrin occlusion, after blood flashback or with a fibrin sleeve, urokinase can be used to clear the catheter. Streptokinase is reserved for the management of serious central vein thrombosis to avoid sensitising the patient.

Catheter damage

The use of connection devices or extension sets reduces the need to clamp the catheter and prolongs catheter life. Repair kits are available if fracture occurs. Subcutaneous ports eventually leak; this becomes apparent when the patient complains of pain around the infusion site. New ports can be attached to the existing catheter.

Effect of PN on other organ systems

Parenteral nutrition may affect such organ systems as the hepatobiliary system, the immune system and the skeleton. Any theoretical detrimental effect must be weighed against the known impairment of organ function associated with the malnutrition that this treatment seeks to prevent or reverse.

Changes in organ function may be a reflection of the underlying disease, malnutrition, drug treatment, and lack of oral or enteral nutrition, as well as the effect of PN. The development of hepatobiliary disease in patients who are treated with prolonged PN illustrates this point. Some forms of hepatobiliary disease occur more commonly in patients with inflammatory bowel disease; the lack of oral nutrition leads to biliary sludge, and possible changes in intestinal permeability with toxin absorption. The administration of excessive amounts of glucose may cause hepatic steatosis, and in neonatal patients the excessive prescription of amino acids has been incriminated in the development of cholestasis. Metabolic bone disease in some patients is attributable to previous malnutrition and exposure to corticosteroid therapy. The influence of PN on bone metabolism is controversial.

RESOURCES FOR PN

The management of PN is enhanced by the presence of a Nutrition Support Team (NST). There should be a programme for staff education and training, especially for doctors, nurses and pharmacists. An audit programme is an essential resource to monitor quality of treatment, costs and complication rates.

The NST may vary in composition and role between different hospitals. Most successful teams will include a nurse specialist in nutrition, a pharmacist, a dietitian, a biochemist and a doctor. There may be more than one team, each representing specific areas within the hospital; for example intensive care, child health, and the medical and surgical floor. The teams will have an interventional role to implement guidelines approved by the nutritional advisory group, consisting of a representative from each of the teams.

Although PN can be undertaken on most wards in adequately equipped hospitals, there is an advantage in confining CPN to parts of the hospital with sufficient experience of this treatment to maintain an adequate standard of expertise and practice.

Home parenteral nutrition should only be undertaken by units with a nutritional support team, and an extensive experience of PN and intestinal failure.

HOME PARENTERAL NUTRITION

Patients considered to be candidates for home parenteral nutrition (HPN) should be referred to centres with the required experience and support facilities. The indication for HPN is permanent intestinal failure. In the UK the most frequent indication for this is short bowel syndrome related to Crohn's disease. In the USA and some European countries AIDS and cancer are common indications, but relatively few of these patients are treated by HPN in the UK. The majority of patients with AIDS and cancer die within a year and more studies are needed to define the role of HPN in these diseases.

Protocols are now readily available for the training of patients and their carers in catheter techniques and in the recognition and management of problems The importance of counselling patients and relatives, as well as the availability of a 24 h telephone contact number for advice, cannot be overstressed.

REFERENCES

Askanazi J, Carpentier YA, Elwyn DH, Nordenstrom J, Jeevanandam M, Rosembaums H et al 1980 Influence of total parenteral nutrition on fuel utilisation in injury and sepsis. Annals of Surgery 191.40–46

Barnett MI, Cosslett AG 1995 Parenteral nutrition formulation. In: Payne-James J, Grimble G, Silk D (eds) Artificial nutrition support in clinical practice. Edward Arnold, London, pp 323–332

British Society of Gastroenterology 1997 Guidelines on artificial nutritional support. British Society of Gastroenterology, London

Burnham WR 1995 The role of the nutrition support team. In: Payne-James J, Grimble G, Silk D (eds) Artificial nutritional support in clinical practice. Edward Arnold, London, pp 175–186

Elia M 1995 Changing concepts of nutrient requirements in disease: implications for artificial nutritional support. Lancet 1:279–1284

Hill GL 1992 Disorders of nutritional metabolism in clinical surgery: understanding management. Churchill Livingstone, Edinburgh

Linares J, Sitges-Sera A, Garaas J et al 1985 Pathogenesis of catheter sepsis: a prospective study with quantitative and semi-quantitative culture of hub and segments. Journal of Clinical Microbiology 21:357–360

Johnston DA, Walker K, Richards J, Pennington CR 1992 Ethanol flush for the prevention of catheter occlusion. Clinical Nutrition 11:97–100

Malone M, Shenkin A, Fell GS, Irving MH 1989 Evaluation of a trace element preparation in patients receiving home parenteral nutrition. Clinical Nutrition 8:307–312

Matuchansky C, Messing B, Jeejeebhoy KN, Beliah M, Allard JP 1992 Cyclical parenteral nutrition, Lancet 340:588–592

Payne-James J, De Gara CJ, Grimble GK, Silk DBA 1995 Artificial nutritional support in hospitals in the United Kingdom – 1994: 3rd National Survey. Clinical Nutrition 14:329–335

Payne-James J, Khawaja HT (1993) First choice for total parenteral nutrition: the peripheral route. Journal of Parenteral and Enteral Nutrition 17:468–471

Pennington CR 1991 Parenteral nutrition: the management of complications. Clinical Nutrition 10.133–137

Pennington CR 1995 Central vein thrombosis during home parenteral nutrition. Clinical Nutrition 14(suppl 1):52–55

Pennington CR (ed) 1996 Current perspectives on parenteral nutrition in adults. British Association for Parenteral and Enteral Nutrition, Maidenhead

Solomon SN, Kirby DS 1990 The refeeding syndrome: a review. Journal of Parenteral and Enteral Nutrition 14:90–95

Tighe MJ, Wong C, Martin IG, McMahon MJ 1996 Do heparin, hydrocortisone, and glyceryl trinitrate influence thrombophlebitis during full intravenous nutrition via a peripheral vein? Journal of Parenteral and Enteral Nutrition 19:507–509.

2

The multidisciplinary team

Jill Hudson

Introduction
Role of the multidisciplinary team
Benefits of a multidisciplinary team

Success of the multidisciplinary team
Summary and recommendations

INTRODUCTION

Methods of providing optimal care for patients requiring artificial nutrition have changed considerably since the introduction of parenteral nutrition (PN) in the 1970s. Initially PN was associated with serious metabolic and catheter-related complications, and was therefore viewed with understandable caution. To ensure appropriate care for patients receiving specialist intravenous nutrition, a new way of managing patient care was needed.

Malnutrition within the healthcare setting is a condition that has been well researched and documented. The multidisciplinary group of healthcare professionals known as the Nutrition Support Team (NST) evolved from the desire to create nutrition as a positive therapy for hospital patients, and so reduce the incidence of morbidity and mortality associated with undernutrition (Taylor & Goodinson-McLaren 1992). The NST provides consultant and specialist services that enable protocols, standards, education, audit and quality assurance to be achieved by the specialist team. The success of this model depends on a director who possesses the organisational skills to ensure that the administrative and clinical functions of the team are coordinated.

In addition to the NST model for the organisation of nutritional support, there is another model known as the Nutrition Support Committee (NSC). In the NSC it is often a physician who is responsible for the patient's nutritional care, while other committee members, e.g. dietitian, nurse and pharmacist, perform identified responsibilities as agreed by the committee. The committee is therefore responsible for the development of protocols, guidelines, in-service education and quality assurance. Although this model carries a lower cost than the NST, it will often take longer to implement and will require an increased awareness and commitment by the medical and nursing staff to provide prompt and appropriate nutrition to the malnourished patient.

Providing nutritional support for the critically ill and malnourished patient demands increased expertise from those healthcare professionals responsible for patient care. Whether or not a formal NST/NSC exists, effective leadership is crucial in the motivation of providing nutrition to the malnourished patient. However, where a NST/NSC does not officially exist, the need for effective communication between healthcare professionals is even more essential.

In both the NST and NSC models, leadership and enthusiasm are important for the successful coordination of the team. Two aspects of leadership vital in a team of this type are the development of patient care and team administration. Generally it is the clinician, knowledgeable in clinical nutrition, who will assume the medical supervision of patients requiring artificial nutrition, whereas it is often the nurse who assumes responsibility for supervising the administration and the day to day clinical function of the NST/NSC.

ROLE OF THE MULTIDISCIPLINARY TEAM

The NST/NSC is a multidisciplinary group of professionals who share a common goal in providing specialist care to patients requiring nutritional support (ASPEN 1990, Matarese & Gottschlich 1998). To achieve such a goal and ensure the team's success, the roles and responsibilities of each team member must be clearly defined (See Table 2.1).

Members of the multidisciplinary team

In most cases the NST/NSC multidisciplinary team consists of the following members:

- consultant clinician
- clinical nurse specialist
- dietitian
- pharmacist.

Additional support from other disciplines is essential to ensure the smooth and safe running of patient care. Additional support is available from the following:

- biochemist
- microbiologist
- infection control clinical nurse specialist
- ward nursing staff
- speech therapist
- psychologist.

Wherever possible, patients should be involved in the decision-making process of nutritional support. This will ensure that patients and their families are well informed of any proposed treatment.

Table 2.1   Observations/actions made by the NST

Team member	Observation/actions
Clinician	Supervises team Communicates with other clinicians Chief prescriber of PN Places central feeding tubes/lines
Clinical nurse specialist	Nutritional assessment Determines venous access Assists with/places peripheral/central line Staff education/liaison Acts as advocate, counsellor and advisor Vitamin and trace element analysis Research
Dietitian	Organises specialised formulae of enteral feed Performs anthropometry/formal nutritional assessment Determines energy/protein requirements Advises re weaning from PN to EN/oral supplements to normal diet
Pharmacist	Aseptic compounding of PN Advises re formulation, plumbing, delivery of PN Advises re drug–nutrient interactions/compatibility of solutions Collates laboratory data
Biochemist	Advises re specific laboratory investigations Vitamin and trace element analysis Interpretation of laboratory data
Microbiologist/ infection nurse	Identifies colonisation of lines Treats cvc sepsis

Table kindly provided by Clare Burnett.

Collective roles

The NST/NSC aims to detect those patients at risk of undernutrition and provide for them the most appropriate therapeutic and cost-effective treatment in a safe and controlled manner. To achieve this, the members of the team each perform an equally important role, which collectively provides an effective and efficient support service. It is to be expected that the ideas and roles of the NST/NSC may overlap and vary slightly from hospital to hospital according to the composition of the team, members' interests and experience, and financial constraints of the Trusts

Individual roles

Consultant clinician

Generally, the consultant clinician within the NST/NSC has an interest in gastroenterology and nutrition, and may function as a gastrointestinal surgeon or gastroenterologist. This role will vary and may include liaison with other clinicians to ensure the existence of good working relationships

(Burnham 1995). Additionally, the clinician's role will often involve taking responsibility for the nutritional care of all patients referred to the NST/ NSC (Hamoui & Nichols 1993). The clinician will also evaluate patho-physiology, predict clinical course, and ensure nutritional goals are met and the appropriate nutritional formulae delivered (Taylor & Goodinson-McLaren 1992).

Historically the clinician has been responsible for the insertion of central venous catheters (cvcs), which have subsequently been cared for by the clinical nurse specialist (CNS) within the team. Alternatively, in some clinical centres this role has been shared or extended to that of the CNS within the team (Hamilton 1995). It is often considered desirable for more than one member of the nursing or medical team to be competent in the insertion of cvcs, as this allows the team to function effectively and efficiently if one member is absent due to sickness, holiday or educational commitments.

Finally, the clinician will often provide the liaison between the team and the hospital board, ensuring that the issue of nutritional support and its funding are addressed at this level.

Clinical nurse specialist

The role of the CNS is a vital, varied and progressive one within any NST/ NSC. It is therefore not uncommon for more than one CNS to be attached to a NST/NSC. The CNS has a unique role and one that often impinges upon other disciplines. Therefore, the CNS requires a relaxed, flexible and sensitive approach to the many responsibilities within the role.

Educational role. The CNS is responsible for setting local protocols of care for the administration of PN and catheter care. Once protocols or guidelines are agreed, it is the responsibility of the CNS to undertake the implementation of such protocols at ward level. This becomes an ongoing process owing to nursing staff turnover and new staff requiring training in all aspects of patient care.

Additionally, it is often the role of the CNS to educate and support nursing colleagues at ward level when new equipment is introduced by the NST/NSC team. Education extends to ward nurses, student nurses, student dietitians and junior medical personnel. In order to cascade information the CNS may also choose to create a link nurse system, electing a nurse mentor from each clinical area, e.g. intensive care, paediatrics, etc., enabling all specialities to keep up to date with modern nutritional methods. This can be an effective method of providing the necessary education if the NSC model is adopted or if the clinical area covers more than one site. Some hospitals are fortunate in having a paediatric CNS, allocated to addressing the nutritional needs of children alone.

The educational role of the nurse within the NST/NSC extends from hospital personnel to patients, relatives and carers of patients referred for home parenteral nutrition (HPN) (Hamoui & Nichols 1993). The CNS is responsible for ensuring that patients requiring HPN are competent, confident and safe to administer HPN independently, in the community. This can be an extremely time-consuming and complex area of the CNS's role. However, once the patient is safely discharged, the sense of achievement in contributing to the safe discharge of a patient receiving HPN is immensely satisfying for both the patient and the nurse.

Clinical role. The clinical role of the CNS is primarily associated with day to day assessment, monitoring, and delivery of PN (Taylor & Goodinson-McLaren 1992). Owing to the regular liaison with staff at ward level, the CNS is often in the best position to receive new referrals and address difficulties related to PN that may arise. This interaction allows the CNS to monitor and facilitate the implementation of appropriate selection protocols. In some cases the CNS will also take on a phlebotomist's role, which ensures that blood results are available for review on the daily NST ward round or the NSC weekly meeting. This role can extend to retrieving blood cultures from the cvc used for the administration of PN if infection of the catheter is suspected. By ensuring that only dedicated personnel harvest blood from the feeding catheter, the risk of catheter contamination is reduced (Grant 1992).

Personnel role. The success of the NST/NSC depends upon coordination and cooperation among team members who respect the contribution of their colleagues. The CNS liaises between all members of the multidisciplinary team and it often falls to the CNS to promote and direct team building.

In addition to ensuring team harmony, the CNS is often the most appropriate discipline to act as the patient's advocate (Silk 1994), conveying the patient's thoughts and feelings to the remaining members of the NST/NSC to guarantee the patient's interests are considered and verbalised (Silk 1994).

Audit. The most critical issue for the survival of the NST/NSC is to demonstrate reduced healthcare costs, reduced patient complications, and improved patient outcomes resulting from the NST/NSC approach. Via the NST/NSC significant savings can be made by appropriate patient selection, prevention of overfeeding, reduced use of non-standard regimens, and general cost analysis that reduces waste.

Audit is therefore an important issue and will encompass many aspects of the service and delivery of PN. It is often the responsibility of the CNS to audit the effectiveness of the team. Areas of audit often include sepsis rate of PN catheters, average length of feeding, metabolic complications, as well as the number of inappropriate referrals to the team. Through the collation of this information the team can reflect upon their progress and detect and target areas where improvements can be made.

Also, through regular liaison at ward level, the CNS becomes the member of the team who usually receives information regarding failed ancillary equipment, PN catheter performance, etc. The CNS can collate this information and liaise with the suppliers of this equipment, ensuring that they are aware of actual and potential failings regarding their products and systems. Additionally, the CNS can liaise with national bodies to ensure that PN and HPN records are regularly updated with relevant information.

Budget. With the implementation of Trust status, the responsibility for coordinating the budget of the nutrition service now often falls to the CNS. However, this will vary from hospital to hospital. Through control of the budget at this level the NST is able not only to evaluate the pharmaceutical products, but also to select the most appropriate and cost-effective equipment to be used for the administration of PN.

Research. Many clinical and laboratory research projects require significant investment in terms of personnel, time and finance, which may not be available to all NST/NSC. However, participation in nursing-related research associated with clinical nutrition is a project often considered worthwhile for the CNS within this speciality.

Dietitian

The dietitian has a vital role within the framework of any NST/NSC. The dietitian is in a position to assess the patient's actual nutritional intake, desired intake and potential nutritional requirements. To achieve this the dietitian must assess the patient accurately whilst considering clinical condition and the implications of nutritional support. Areas to be addressed include:

1. assessing the patient on an individual basis; and
2. establishing a profile of the patient's nutritional requirements with relation to such issues as:
   • general condition and mobility;
   • weight loss/weight gain;
   • gastrointestinal function;
   • awareness of compliance difficulties;
   • liaison with medical staff to assess the predicted duration before gastrointestinal function is restored;
   • knowledge of alternative sources of nutrition;
   • individual nutritional and fluid requirements;
   • patient preference and previous experiences;
   • patient's 'normal' dietary intake and food preferences;
   • psychological state.

Once the dietitian has collated this information the nutritional requirements of the patient can be translated into a formula which may then be understood and utilised by the other team members (Hamoui & Nichols 1993). By assessing the patient in this manner the dietitian is able to advise on the introduction of the most appropriate method of providing nutrition, increase enteral nutrition intake, and maximise absorption by the intestine. However, when the use of the gut is contraindicated the dietitian will also provide advice on the patient's requirements via the parenteral route.

Monitoring of patients. Once the need for nutritional support has been established, the dietitian contributes to the monitoring of hospital- and community-based patients requiring PN (Taylor & Goodinson-McLaren 1992). Monitoring will include weight, muscle tone, energy intake and, in discussion with other team members, interpretation of blood results. In addition to routine monitoring of biochemistry and haematology, trace elements and vitamins are also considered.

With the continuous assessment of patients the dietitian can advise on the timing of the transition from PN to enteral nutrition (EN). Wherever possible it is advisable for the dietitian to continue to care for and advise patients on methods to increase enteral intake until gastrointestinal function is considered 'normal' and a full enteral diet becomes possible. For patients receiving long-term PN it is the dietitian's responsibility to adjust the individual patient's energy requirements when the clinical condition demands a change in requirements.

Ongoing support. The dietitian has a strong commitment to the support and education of patients, relatives, nursing staff, medical staff and students. Patients requiring artificial nutrition often suffer psychological and emotional difficulties with the manipulation or possible exclusion of their diet. Within this context it is important that the dietitian develops an effective rapport with patients requiring nutritional support over a long period of time. Many patients will experience difficulties when EN is implemented after a long period on PN and show no interest in food. Dietitians are often well placed to advise patients in selecting suitable, small quantities of food and can help them to overcome fears and anxieties associated with eating after a period of abstinence.

Pharmacist

The NST/NSC pharmacist is an expert on the subject of compounding nutritional formulation and will be instrumental in the aseptic production of the patient's requirements. The role of the pharmacist is an important one and often underestimated, as the majority of the pharmacist's work is conducted behind the scenes. As with the other team members, the role of the pharmacist can be divided into three main categories: clinical issues, patient monitoring and research/education.

Clinical issues. Clinically, the pharmacist is involved in consultation with other team members regarding the PN formula. The pharmacist is responsible for anticipating any drug–nutrient interaction. Once the formula is agreed, the pharmacist will be in a position to review the compatibility of all the components and ensure the clinical stability of the nutritional formula.

The pharmacist is also responsible for compounding PN. To enable a department to compound PN the pharmacy department must gain a licence from the Medical Control Agency, who act to ensure that the infusion is compounded in a safe and aseptic manner. The formula is compounded by the pharmacist and his team under sterile conditions before the product is available for infusion. The pharmacist is also responsible for the storage, packing and transportation of PN, thus ensuring its arrival in a safe and controlled manner. In some departments the compounding of PN occurs on the day of use. To achieve this, the pharmacist must review the patient's biochemical status on a daily basis and liaise with medical personnel to ensure an appropriate formula and volume is prescribed to meet the patient's clinical needs.

Any queries regarding the prescription and the supply and replacement of PN in an emergency will be attended to by the on-call pharmacist. However, to supply PN out of hours is both expensive and often unnecessary and should only occur when alternative arrangements cannot be made.

Patient monitoring. As with other team members, the pharmacist has a responsibility to ensure that each patient is monitored closely (Silk 1994). The main monitoring responsibility for the pharmacist is the analysis of serum biochemistry, fluid balance and potential drug interactions in relation to the individual patient's clinical condition.

Educational role. The pharmacist has a wealth of knowledge and therefore has a responsibility to educate other disciplines as well as patients and their families regarding PN. This may include advising on suggested enteral preparations that the patient may find more tolerable than administration of a parenteral preparation. With regard to patients receiving HPN, the pharmacist has a responsibility to liaise closely with commercial pharmaceutical companies who provide nutrients to patients in the community, ensuring the transition from hospital to home is as smooth as possible.

Referral to the NST/NSC

It is important that the referral system to the NST/NSC is uncomplicated, allowing a variety of disciplines, e.g. ward nurses, ward dietitians, pharmacists, speech therapists and junior doctors, to gain advice and guidance on the patient's nutritional requirements and subsequent care. Each referral must be considered on an individual basis by the multidisciplinary team.

BENEFITS OF A MULTIDISCIPLINARY TEAM

The benefits of a NST/NSC are three-fold and include:

• clinical benefits

- financial benefits
- education/research benefits.

Clinical benefits

The major benefit of a NST or NSC is the ability to assess accurately the patient's nutritional state (Reynolds 1995). Nutritional support for the patient may be in the form of EN or PN, depending on the patient's requirements and potential gastrointestinal function. Once the patient is receiving nutritional support, the NST/NSC is able to monitor progress and adjust therapy as required. The reported benefits of a NST have been highlighted by BAPEN (Silk 1994). Evidence provided by BAPEN (Silk 1994) suggests that there is clinical improvement in wound healing, immune response and muscle strength in patients receiving artificial nutrition as prescribed and monitored by a NST.

Specific clinical benefits of a NST/NSC in association with PN are described below.

Reduced catheter complications

With a dedicated person from the NST inserting and maintaining catheters for the administration of PN, the rate of catheter insertion complications, catheter sepsis and subsequent catheter-related complications is dramatically reduced (Silk 1994, Burnham 1995, Hamilton 1995). Additionally, Traeger et al (1986) note that catheter-related complications are less serious if venous access is gained and managed by the nurse representative within the NST (see Ch. 9).

Reduced metabolic and mechanical complications

With the intravenous administration of a highly complex and sophisticated nutritional feed, mechanical and metabolic complications become inevitable as a result of the effect of artificial nutrition on principal organs involved in the metabolism of PN. However, regular monitoring of the patient receiving PN by the NST means that complications can be promptly recognised and addressed. Through the expertise of the team, the NST is able to anticipate problems and thus avoid them. Additionally, the NST/NSC can review and implement the most appropriate, safe and cost-effective apparatus to be used for the administration of PN for both hospital- and community-based patients.

Financial benefits

The administration of PN is an expensive and time-consuming therapy within the hospital setting. The most critical task for the NST/NSC is to demonstrate reduced costs, reduced complications and improved patient outcomes due to team intervention and creativity.

Specific areas include:

1. A reduction in the incidence of catheter-related sepsis. Reduced mechanical and metabolic complications and increased patient wellbeing results in the average length of hospital stay being shortened, thus reducing the cost of treatment (Silk 1994, Burnham 1995).

2. With careful selection and assessment the most effective and appropriate form of nutritional support is prescribed (Burnham 1995).

3. Significant cost savings can be realised by the experienced NST through standardising preparations, reducing the use of non-standard preparations, and performing cost analysis of supplies and preparations to determine which products provide the best value for money. In addition, owing to the experience of an established NST/NSC fewer laboratory investigations will be necessary, therefore reducing costs in this area.

Education/research benefits

Through its expertise and specific knowledge the NST/NSC becomes a resource to other disciplines by providing research-based information and ideas. This may then be cascaded to healthcare colleagues in a variety of settings who may benefit from evidence-based nutritional advice from the NST/NSC.

SUCCESS OF THE MULTIDISCIPLINARY TEAM

The success of the NST/NSC is vital for the future of the service. This is dependent on four areas:

- direction of the team
- communication
- motivation of team members
- formal evidence of the team's success.

Direction of the team

The NST/NSC must identify a person to lead or act as director of the team to highlight the short- and long-term goals of the service. For the NST/NSC team to operate it must market its service to medical teams who can then confidently refer patients for prompt nutritional assessment, subsequent therapy and successful patient outcomes. Respect from the referring medical teams can only be gained by the team becoming accessible and working with clinicians to build and maintain their support. Without clear direction, team members will work in isolation and ultimately pull in opposite directions. This will rapidly become apparent to both the patients and those who make use of the service.

Motivation of team members

Due to the current economic climate within the Health Service, many administrators do not fully appreciate the importance of providing nutritional support for patients. To demonstrate the benefits and accomplishments achieved by the NST/NSC it is vital for the team to remain united and adopt a creative approach. Lack of motivation within the NST/NSC can result in reduced standards of patient care, which will have a demoralising effect on both the patients and the medical and nursing teams caring for them. Alimo-Metcalfe (1994) has shown that motivating factors such as autonomy and the provision of challenging and interesting work have long-lasting motivational effects in the workplace. Therefore, the encouragement of team members to follow personal interests and develop themselves through education and short-term projects, whilst integrating ideas into the total aims of the NST/NSC, will aid in promoting team enthusiasm.

Auditing is an essential indicator of the NST/NSC and will enable team members to recognise trends that, once identified, can be addressed. Through identifying improvements in patient care the NST/NSC will be encouraged and stimulated to succeed.

Communication

Effective communication based on mutual respect and a commitment to collaborative practice is vital for the continuing success of the NST/NSC (Taylor & Goodison-McLaren 1992). Without appropriate patient referrals, the service will ultimately fail.

It is essential that the team meets regularly to discuss PN patient-related problems and the focus of the team. All team members must be aware of the extent of their role and recognise their limitations and the boundaries of their input. This in turn will aid in avoiding professional territorialism and conflict within the team (Taylor & Goodison-McLaren 1992).

Definition of roles is especially crucial as roles within the team develop and change. For example, the role of the CNS is expanding out of recognition with the development of nurse education and expansion of skills that nurses are able to acquire, such as central line insertion and phlebotomy roles. Without negotiation and clarification other team members may feel threatened and become defensive about their value in the team, instead of maximising enthusiasm and expertise to achieve prime patient care.

Formal evidence of the team's success

The NST/NSC needs to become vocal in its accomplishments, particularly when these enhance the organisational image (Matarese & Gottschlich 1998). To maintain the NST/NSC purchasers must be aware of the team's success. This can be communicated through publishing the success rate of reducing complications, highlighting the number of appropriate referrals and the reduced number of bed days due to prompt and effective nutritional support, with the significant associated savings in cost.

In the economic climate of today's Health Service, improved quality of care in association with reduced expenditure will not fail to impress purchasers of the continuing need for a NST/NSC.

SUMMARY AND RECOMMENDATIONS

Establishing priorities for the allocation of healthcare resources will continue to present difficulties in terms of funding. The challenge continues in the justification of allocating sufficient resources for the detection, assessment and subsequent management of the malnourished patient. Nutritional support prescribed by a NST/NSC for malnourished patients has proven clinical benefit (Silk 1994). Where possible it is preferable for hospitals to provide the expertise of a NST/NSC to offer support and advice on the management of the malnourished patient. It is evident that not all centres have the benefit of a dedicated NST or NSC. Therefore, nursing and medical personnel cannot rely on the expertise of others or ignore malnutrition but must become proactive in seeking and developing their own methods of implementing nutritional care for patients. Support groups such as BAPEN are available for all disciplines to use and obtain knowledge from. Where a NST or NSC is available, the team provide a united and motivated approach to supplying up to date information and support to patients and colleagues. In this way malnutrition can be made a condition of the past within a hospital setting.

REFERENCES

Alimo-Metcalfe B 1994 The poverty of PRP. Health Service Journal: October 20:22–24
ASPEN (American Society for Parenteral and Enteral Nutrition) 1990 Nutrition Support Team resource kit, pp 1–23. ASPEN, Silver Spring, MD
Burnham WR 1995 The role of a Nutritional Support Team. In: Payne-James J, Grimble G, Silk D (eds) Artificial nutritional support in clinical practice. Edward Arnold, London
Grant JP 1992 Handbook of total parenteral nutrition, 2nd edn. WB Saunders, Philadelphia
Hamilton H 1995 Central lines inserted by clinical nurse specialists. Nursing Times 91(17):38–39
Hamoui E, Nichols SLO 1993 The Nutritional Support Team: organisation and dynamics. In: Rombeau JL, Caldwell MD (eds) Clinical nutrition: parenteral nutrition, 2nd edn. WB Saunders, London, ch. 14

Matarese LE, Gottschlich MM 1998 Contemporary nutritional support practice – a clinical guide. WB Saunders, Philadelphia, ch 1, pp 3–13

Reynolds N, McWhirter JP, Pennington CR 1995 Nutritional support teams: an integral part of developing a gastroenterological service. Gut 37(6): 740–742

Silk D (ed). 1994 Organisation of nutrition support in hospitals. BAPEN, Maidenhead

Taylor S, Goodinson-McLaren S 1992 Nutritional support: a team approach. Wolfe Publishing, London

Traeger SM, Williams GB, Milliren G, Young DS, Fisher M, Haug III MT 1986 Total parenteral nutrition by a Nutrition Support Team: improved quality of care. Journal of Parenteral and Enteral Nutrition 10(4):408–412

3

Patient assessment

Clare Burnett

Introduction
Bedside nutritional assessment
Assessment of gastrointestinal function
Parenteral versus enteral nutrition
Referral for PN

Considerations for PN in specific disease
   processes
Peripheral parenteral nutrition
Summary

INTRODUCTION

Food is vital for living.

I eat to live, to serve and also if it so happens to enjoy, but I do not eat for the sake of enjoyment.

(Mohandas Mahatma Gandhi, 1869–1948)

One should eat to live not live to eat.

(Jean Baptiste Molière, 1622–1673, from *Don Juan*)

Nutrition is an essential element for health. There is no disease or illness state that benefits from malnutrition. Traditionally, healthcare professionals within the hospital setting provide for the sick, yet it is within such establishments that malnutrition in patients may go unnoticed. These 'skeletons in the cupboard' may represent as many as 40–50% of adult patients (McWhirter & Pennington 1994). Children are also afflicted, with undernutrition a frequently reported occurrence in hospital in the acute setting, in intensive care and in children with chronic illness (Moy et al 1990).

These factors provide 'food for thought' as to how the nurse may recognise vulnerable individuals through accurate assessment of nutritional state, and thus recommend them for appropriate nutritional support. This chapter aims to provide information to help nurses develop these skills.

BEDSIDE NUTRITIONAL ASSESSMENT

A nutritional assessment may be undertaken by a trained nurse, a dietitian or a clinician. A trained nurse is ideally placed to perform a simple bedside nutritional assessment. The nurse is able to take an accurate history and use skills of observation and touch as part of the relationship as primary carer. There is no one accurate assessment tool that may be utilised to define nutritional status. Nutritional assessment tends to be coupled with a metabolic assessment, the latter including assessment of body fluid and

---

Box 3.1 Bedside nutritional assessment

Assessment = Nutritional assessment + Metabolic assessment
↓ ↓

Height and weight	Serum protein assays
Anthropometry	Biochemical indices
Skin	Fluid and electrolyte balance
Body temperature	
Nails	
Hair	
Mood	

---

electrolytes and endocrine homeostasis (Box 3.1). Within a Nutrition Support Team (NST) metabolic assessment should be the role of a trained clinician.

Why perform a bedside nutritional assessment

Malnutrition is the depletion of essential nutrients and loss of body/tissue stores. Its development may be of rapid onset if intervention is not sought. It is associated with a declining spiral of events that results in death. A nutritional assessment should:

1. identify those already suffering from malnutrition
2. identify those at risk of malnutrition
3. encourage early referral for nutritional support
4. evaluate the effect of nutritional support.

Malnutrition is linked to increased morbidity and mortality. There is a causal relationship between malnutrition and a diminished host immune response, increasing vulnerability to infection. Higher depression scores and apathy are reported in association with weight loss (Lennard Jones 1992), with fatigue and impaired concentration demonstrated as additional clinical signs. There is loss of muscle bulk and generalised decrease in muscle function causing compromise to body systems such as the cardiac and respiratory systems.

Malnutrition has serious implications for recovery from illness and general health with an associated increase in length of hospital stay for such patients. Therefore, prevention of malnutrition and the provision of appropriate nutritional support is vital in order to improve clinical outcome and reduce costs of healthcare.

How to perform a bedside nutritional assessment

This can be achieved through accurate history taking and skills of clinical observation (Box 3.2).

Box 3.2   Summary of bedside nutritional assessment

Observation
- Weight and height (always on admission to hospital)
- BMI
- Hand grip
- Hair, teeth, gums and skin
- Pulse and blood pressure
- Body temperature
- Nitrogen balance
- Fluid balance

History taking
- Physiological: – poor appetite
                  – nausea and vomiting
                  – pain, diarrhoea, constipation
- Psychological: depression, phobia, unhappiness
- Social: finances, mobility, culture and religion
- Drug and alcohol intake

History taking

A detailed dietary history is important as part of a nursing assessment. A food diary may quantify food intake. Pertinent questions should be asked regarding meal size and their frequency, changes in appetite and taste and avoidance of specific foods. The patient should be considered in a holistic manner. From a physiological perspective, consideration should be given to anorexia, diarrhoea, nausea and vomiting, pain or constipation. From a psychological stand, depression, phobia or adverse life events should be considered. From a social perspective, financial restraints, poor mobility and impact of cultural or religious beliefs should be considered. Drugs and alcohol intake markedly affect nutritional state and this needs to be ascertained through sensitive questioning. Food and drugs interact in many ways. Those with a history of long-term use of medication/drug therapy may be at risk of drug-induced nutritional deficiencies. Alcohol in particular may cause wasting that is chronic in nature with altered micronutrient state, e.g. of vitamins and minerals.

Clinical observation

Height and weight. Accurate measurements of height and body weight are the prerequisite of nutritional assessment. Scales, preferably electronic, should be correctly calibrated. Weight loss is a clinical sign of negative energy and protein balance. Weight loss of >10% of pre-illness weight is clinically significant and weight loss of 10–20% is associated with functional abnormalities and a poor clinical outcome, especially in surgical patients (Sitges-Serra et al 1990).

Misinterpretation of body weight may occur in the presence of dehydration, oedema and ascites (Klein et al 1997). Observation of the patient and assessment of his hydration status will identify these states. Further observation will reveal wasting of muscle mass, especially around the buttocks; a thin face with marked cheek bones; and prominent bones, especially the ribs and scapula. Anthropometry using skinfold thickness and mid upper arm circumference is a useful tool to determine body fat and muscle bulk. However, this requires an experienced operator and is subject to some unreliability in the presence of oedema. Routine anthropometry is of great use in the patient requiring long-term nutritional intervention.

Body height/length is performed using calibrated scales or a board. In children, height is used in conjunction with body weight and compared with age on specific centile charts. This is an imperative measurement as discrepancies in a child's growth may indicate a chronic failure to thrive or underlying chronic illness.

Calculation of body mass index (BMI) provides an additional useful tool when assessing for malnutrition. Nomograms are available to assist in calculation and represent the normal limits. A BMI of <20 kg/m^2 suggests possible malnutrition and values < 18 suggest likely malnutrition (Norton 1996). The following formula is used to calculate BMI:

$$BMI = \frac{mass\ in\ kg}{(height\ in\ m)^2}$$

Measurement of head circumference is included as part of the child's assessment. The younger the child, the more vulnerable he is to the adversity of poor nutrition. A child under 2 years is particularly vulnerable in terms of the growing and developing brain, an organ that attains almost adult capacity by the age of 2 years. Head circumference measurements are plotted according to age on centile charts for the child under 2 years.

Strength and muscle bulk. This is adversely affected by a poor nutritional state. The patient may have a poor hand grip and altered mobility. Apathy with ease of fatigue may present as a patient complaint.

Hair and skin. Hair should be observed for signs of alopecia, dullness and thinning. Similarly the skin is also susceptible due to rapid cell turnover of epithelial tissue. Skin should be observed for pallor, dryness, for bruising, infection, pressure sores and evidence of delayed healing. Nutritional deficiencies may be evident in teeth and gums, which should be observed for evidence of decay, bleeding and ulceration. Examination of the eyes may reveal pale conjunctivae. There may be evidence of lesions around the mouth such as angular chelitis and the tongue may be pale or discoloured.

Additional measurements. Having obtained accurate measurements of height and weight, pulse, blood pressure and core body temperature should be measured. Significant malnutrition results in a reduced metabolic rate and a compensatory lowered body temperature. Significant reduction in body fat reduces the thermoinsulatory protection for the body and creates a heightened sensitivity to cold. A 24 h urine collection for nitrogen balance should be considered, especially in the presence of diarrhoea, vomiting and protein loss from exuding wounds. This will enable accurate assessment of the individual patient's protein requirements.

ASSESSMENT OF GASTROINTESTINAL FUNCTION

Assessment of gut function is necessary in order to determine appropriate nutritional support. This may become an additional component of the bedside nutritional assessment. The assessment involves the function of the gastrointestinal (GI) tract, from the mouth to the anus. Any dysfunction at any part of the GI tract may hinder the ability to eat and affect the absorption, digestion and excretion of foodstuffs.

Mouth and upper GI tract

Observe the mouth for sores, ulcers and infections such as candida. Poorly fitting or absent dentures in the elderly impede eating. Painful mucositis occurring as a side-effect of cytotoxic drug administration and acquired immune deficiency syndrome (AIDS) may affect the whole of the GI tract and may inhibit a patient from taking any nutrition by mouth. Dysphagia may occur secondary to a cerebrovascular event or carcinoma and stricture of the oesophagus. Achalasia, dyspepsia and gastro-oesophageal reflux (GOR) also adversely affect food ingestion and tolerance.

Stomach and small bowel

Pain is an effect of a number of disease processes creating anorexia and a fear of eating. Crohn's disease is accompanied by wasting, diarrhoea, malabsorption of micronutrients and abdominal pain. Peptic ulcer disease, gastritis, carcinoma of the stomach and small bowel obstruction are a few of many diseases of the upper GI tract that adversely affect nutrient intake.

Large bowel

Diseases of the colon include ulcerative colitis or infectious colitis and symptoms are of pain, diarrhoea and weight loss. The presence of constipation and/or diarrhoea may indicate the presence of carcinoma of the bowel or subacute intestinal obstruction. These are a few of many diseases of the large bowel that may prevent the adequate intake and absorption of nutrients.

Assessment of GI tract function should include:

- accurate fluid balance
- record of intake and output, e.g. from nasogastric tube, fistula etc.
- record of nausea and/or vomiting
- scored pain and relevance to eating
- appetite
- frequency, colour and consistency of stools
- presence of bowel sounds/flatus
- presence of abdominal distension.

Following an assessment of gut function a decision is made as to the most appropriate method of nutritional intervention. The nutritional intervention may be PN or enteral nutrition (EN), and the decision is made jointly by members of the multidisciplinary team or, ideally, by a NST.

The decision focuses around a common philosophy:

If the gut works – use it.

PARENTERAL VERSUS ENTERAL NUTRITION

Enteral nutrition

Enteral nutrition is defined as the provision of liquid formula diets by tube or by mouth into the GI tract. Enteral nutrition has been used with increasing frequency in both the hospital and home setting. It is easy to use and cost-effective in terms of preventing and treating the costly consequences of malnutrition.

The GI tract may be accessed for enteral feeding in a number of ways:

- nasogastric tube
- nasoduodenal tube
- nasojejunal tube
- percutaneous endoscopic/ultrasonographic gastrostomy tube (PEG/PUG) or gastrostomy button
- gastrostomy-jejunal tube
- duodenostomy tube
- jejunostomy tube.

Enteral feeding is the preferred method of feeding patients. However, it may not always be tolerated at levels required to meet the patient's nutritional needs. In this situation, every attempt must be made to deliver at least some nutrition via the GI tract. This ensures the potent trophic effect that luminal nutrition has on gut mucosa. If the GI tract cannot be used safely and effectively, then PN should be implemented or used complementary to enteral feeding. The advantages and disadvantages of enteral feeding are summarised in Box 3.3.

```
Box 3.3   Advantages and disadvantages of enteral feeding

Advantages
• Safe
• Cost-effective
• Trophic effect on GI mucosa
• Avoidance of complications associated with PN
• Socially more acceptable, e.g. gastrostomy button

Disadvantages
• Poor tolerance, e.g. of nasogastric tube
• Diarrhoea/vomiting
• Tube displacement
• Metabolic complications
```

Parenteral nutrition

Parenteral nutrition remains relatively new in the world of medicine. It has come a long way since some of the earliest descriptions of infusing fresh milk into the veins of patients in the late nineteenth century (Hodder 1873, Thomas 1878). Research and experimentation have ensured that modern PN is a safe and often life-saving therapy.

Parenteral nutrition is by no means without complications (see Box 3.4), hence patient selection is specific and demands the attention of a skilled and knowledgeable NST.

```
Box 3.4   Advantages and disadvantages of PN

Advantages
• Provision of life-saving nutritional support
• Guaranteed provision of protein, fat, electrolytes, trace elements and vitamins

Disadvantages
• Complications associated with catheter
• Metabolic complications
• Cost
```

Patient selection for parenteral nutrition

The following categories of patient may be selected for PN:

• patients in whom enteral feeding has failed
• patients in whom enteral feeding is insufficient to meet the nutrient/ fluid demands
• patients in whom a reduced oral intake or nil by mouth status shall exist for more than 5 days*

---

*An adult requirement of 5% dextrose will provide only 500 kcal/day as glucose, no protein, and no vitamins, minerals or trace elements. It is of little nutritional benefit.

- patients with massive small bowel resection
- patients with impaired intestinal motility and/or absorption of nutrients
- premature neonates with immature gut function.

The algorithm shown in Figure 3.1 can be used to reach a decision as to the best method of feeding.

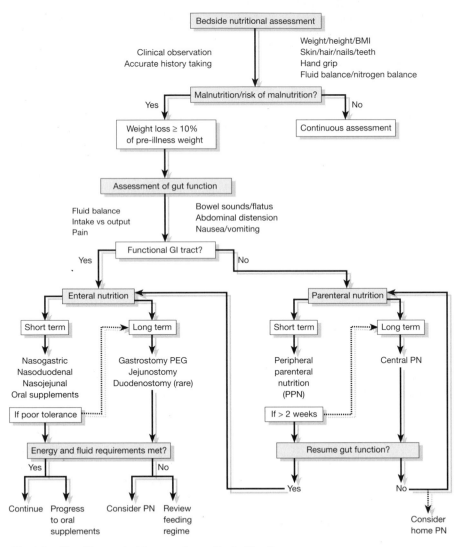

Fig. 3.1 Algorithm to decide upon the method of feeding.

REFERRAL FOR PN

Since the proposals forwarded by the Kings Fund Report of 1992 (Lennard Jones 1992), many more hospitals have developed NSTs. As described in Chapter 2, the NST is a multidisciplinary organisation to which patients are referred for advice and support regarding the management of nutritional status. The NST is often led by a clinician. However, in some hospitals, the specialist nutrition nurse(s) coordinates the organisation of the team. This includes the writing of protocols/guidelines, the setting of standards, staff and patient education, audit and research.

The bedside nutritional assessment and assessment of gut function may reveal a state of nutritional vulnerability and impending/actual malnutrition. It is at this point that a referral should be made to the NST. A referral is made to any member of the NST, often the specialist nurse owing to the close liaison with wards and staff. NSTs meet on a regular basis and it is at one of these meetings that a formal assessment of the patient's nutritional state is made and an appropriate method of feeding implemented. In the absence of a NST, a referral for nutritional support is made to a dietitian who coordinates the type, method and monitoring of nutritional support. Referrals for nutritional support, whether parenteral or enteral, come from a number of areas within a hospital, notably surgery, oncology and neurology.

As a trained nurse making a referral to the NST, the following information is helpful:

1. diagnosis
2. brief medical history
3. bedside nutritional assessment and assessment of gut function
4. patient's admission weight and height and history of weight loss
5. impending surgery/procedures, etc.
6. accurate fluid balance – history of vomiting/diarrhoea.

CONSIDERATIONS FOR PN IN SPECIFIC DISEASE PROCESSES

There are specific indications for the instigation of parenteral feeding. Similarly, there are specific considerations to be made according to the individual patient and his or her presenting complaint. It is imperative to assess each patient *individually* in order to ensure safe nutritional management and prevent complications of feeding that may ensue.

Considerations for the following disease processes are examined in brief:

- short bowel syndrome
- pancreatitis
- gastrointestinal surgery

- inflammatory bowel disease
- gastrointestinal fistula
- malignancy
- acquired immune deficiency syndrome (AIDS)
- burns/sepsis/trauma
- diseases in pregnancy.

Short bowel syndrome

'Short bowel syndrome' is the primary indication for long-term or home PN. It is characterised by malabsorption, dehydration, electrolyte imbalance and a spiral towards malnutrition. Mortality and morbidity are high but dependent upon the length and function of gut remaining, age and preoperative condition of the patient. Such massive surgical resection of bowel is required for:

- volvulus
- infarction of bowel due to occlusion of a major blood vessel
- multiple resections of inflammatory bowel, e.g. Crohn's disease.

The actual length of the adult bowel is controversial in spite of attempts at measurement, both surgically and radiologically. However, the consensus is a bowel length of approximately 300–800 cm with a wide variation according to individuals. Short bowel syndrome relates to the percentage of the total bowel that is removed, but also to the length and quality of the bowel that remains.

It is the small bowel that is responsible for the uptake of nutrients and bile salts. Patients with a small bowel resection of up to 50% often maintain their nutritional state without long-term PN. Patients with a resection of 75%, however, will require long-term PN (ASPEN Board of Directors 1993). Patients with less than 100 cm of small bowel remaining usually require long-term PN (Klein et al 1997). The presence of the ileocaecal valve is an important consideration as this holds important properties of absorption without which severe diarrhoea ensues.

Aggressive enteral feeding may eliminate the need for PN in some patients with short bowel. This should be seriously considered by the NST and attempted if appropriate. In addition, oral/tube rehydration therapy may be used to prevent the need for parenteral fluid replacement. Close attention is made in monitoring fluid and electrolyte balance in the patient with short bowel. The limited absorption of specific nutrients should be considered, for example, fat- and water-soluble vitamins, especially vitamin B_{12}, all minerals and trace elements.

Patients with short bowel syndrome may present as severely malnourished. In this situation all abnormal biochemistry should be corrected prior to artificial feeding and the dietitian then carefully calculates the energy/protein requirements of the individual. The danger here is to over-feed and create a surplus of nutrients that 'overload' the body's suppressed metabolic pathways.

Pancreatitis

Pancreatitis is an inflammatory disease process that has multiple aetiology (see Box 3.5) and presents on a continuum from mild to severe. The majority of pancreatitis presents as acute, mild or moderate, often resolves within 1 week and does not require aggressive nutritional intervention. Indeed, the introduction of nutritional intervention in this group of patients proves to have no effect upon clinical outcome (Klein et al 1997).

Severe acute pancreatitis, however, is characterised by increased meta-bolic demands and a great potential for the development of malnutrition. Severe pancreatitis may be haemorrhagic or necrotising and accom-panied by complications such as pancreatic fistula, pseudocyst and abscess formation. These patients often have protracted periods of limited oral intake owing to multiple surgical manoeuvres, potential admission to intensive care and a prolonged hospital stay. Oral feeding stimulates the inflamed and diseased pancreas, causing severe abdominal pain that may require opiate analgesia.

Traditionally, parenteral nutrition has been utilised as a primary therapy in severe pancreatitis, for the provision of nutrients whilst avoiding pancreatic stimulation. However, a more recent approach has favoured the use of an enteral route.

Jejunostomy feeding has been shown to have a negligible stimulating effect upon the pancreas and is a serious consideration for the patient with acute severe pancreatitis (McClave et al 1997). This is more cost-effective and avoids the potential complications of catheter-related sepsis and meta-bolic imbalance associated with long-term PN. However, jejunal feeding may be abandoned if it proves insufficient to supply the necessary energy requirements or if the patient deteriorates, whereupon parenteral feeding is considered.

Nursing considerations for the patient with severe acute pancreatitis are to closely observe fluid and electrolyte balance. In addition, the nurse

---

Box 3.5   Aetiology of pancreatitis

- Idiopathic
- Gallstones
- Ethanol toxicity
- Chemically induced
- Trauma
- Viral
- Familial variants – rare

should record any fistula output, diarrhoea, vomiting and nasogastric aspirate. Pain is a significant symptom of pancreatitis and needs regular assessment. Increasing pain may signify a deterioration in current state. This may be in relation to commencing oral intake. Consideration should also be made to a misplaced or redirected feeding jejunostomy tube, stimulating the pancreas through accidental feeding higher in the GI tract.

Vitamins and minerals should be closely monitored by the NST, especially with a history of alcohol intake that is often accompanied by low B complex vitamins. Blood glucose should be frequently monitored for hyperglycaemia. Insulin requirements are greater in pancreatitis and the patient may require the administration of sliding-scale insulin, especially if receiving parenteral glucose. Blood samples that return lipaemic should be noted and discussed with the NST. The administration of intravenous lipid, although usually well tolerated, is sometimes poorly so in patients with pancreatitis. Serum triglycerides should be monitored by the NST and alterations made accordingly to the feeding regime. Twenty-four hour collections of urine are beneficial to calculate protein loss and/or balance. Routine nursing observations are essential to aid assessment of the patient's clinical condition.

Gastrointestinal surgery

It is well known that patients who undergo major surgery are at a greater risk of malnutrition than most. This is as a direct cause of the increased metabolic rate and the stress associated with surgery (Eddington et al 1997).

Not surprisingly, patients, females especially, who experience GI surgery are most at risk of malnutrition (Eddington et al 1997, Larsson et al 1995). The majority of patients undergoing GI surgery do not require artificial nutritional support and are suitable for the early introduction of high-energy oral supplements.

Nutritional support in the postoperative period is widely recognised to enhance certain indices of nutritional state: body weight, serum albumin, nitrogen balance and intracellular levels of electrolytes. However, advantages in the route of feeding, i.e. enteral versus parenteral, remain unclear. Parenteral nutrition in the postoperative period has been linked to reports of heightened complications (Klein et al 1997). If the GI tract may be accessed for enteral feeding, this is the preferred route. Indeed, the advent of more sophisticated routes of enteral feeding and the variety of solutions used may see a decrease in the use of PN, especially for major oesophageal or upper GI tract surgery. If EN is not possible, then parenteral feeding is instituted to prevent the onset of starvation and its associated delay in recovery from surgery.

Nursing considerations include documentation of accurate fluid balance. Close monitoring may provide indicators of poor tolerance of enteral feeding, e.g. abdominal distension, nausea and vomiting, large nasogastric aspirates, etc. For the patient receiving PN, nursing considerations include the early detection of potential complications associated with parenteral feeding.

Inflammatory bowel disease

Inflammatory bowel disease (IBD) refers to Crohn's disease and idiopathic ulcerative colitis. IBD is characterised by abdominal pain, diarrhoea and weight loss. Patients suffering IBD are at significant risk of malnutrition due to:

- decreased oral intake
- malabsorption, e.g. of micronutrients
- drug–nutrient interactions
- protein-losing enteropathy
- increased metabolic rate.

Children with IBD may have short stature, poor weight gain and delayed pubertal development. The introduction of EN, either orally or via a feeding tube, in children with IBD promotes growth in terms of body height and weight. Assessment of micronutrient state is important in both adults and children as deficiencies have a marked effect upon many aspects of growth and development, for example tissue healing, muscle function, sight, bones and teeth, and in maintaining intracellular homeostasis.

Traditionally, PN and bowel rest were used as primary therapy for an acute exacerbation of Crohn's disease. Many studies have since shown that the use of defined enteral feeding has a similar outcome to PN in terms of obtaining clinical remission of the disease and supporting nutritional state. The use of elemental diets in the management of Crohn's disease has been shown to be as effective as steroid therapy in inducing short-term remission. Such remission rates are reported to be as high as 60%. However, oral elemental formula is often unpalatable and poorly tolerated by some patients. This affects compliance of treatment and thus clinical outcome. Some patients may require the insertion of an enteral feeding tube to ensure effective delivery of elemental diet.

Ulcerative colitis has a reduced response to dietary manipulation and treatment although nutritional therapy is still of importance in preventing nutritional deficiencies and preserving body mass. PN is considered in patients with ulcerative colitis who are undergoing surgery or whose requirements are unable to be met with EN alone.

Gastrointestinal fistulae

Parenteral nutrition is considered in patients with gastrointestinal fistulae, secondary to Crohn's disease. Nutritional support in patients with gastro-intestinal fistulae improves clinical outcome. Fistulae are characterised by high fluid and electrolyte losses with the risk of generalised peritonitis. Spontaneous closure of the fistula may take considerable time and is often not maintained after the reintroduction of a normal diet. In this time, the patient may have a greatly restricted oral intake and an associated reduction in taste, feelings of hunger and the psychosocial pleasures that accompany eating food.

Patients with IBD may, therefore, be selected for PN, especially in the presence of gastrointestinal fistula, impending surgery or when EN is un-able to meet the patient's nutritional needs. Nursing considerations for the patient with IBD include regular and accurate measurement of weight, fluid, electrolyte and nitrogen balance, especially in patients with gastro-intestinal fistula. If possible, enteral feeding is instigated, even in small amounts, for its trophic effect upon gut mucosa, and oral feeding for its benefit to the patient's psychological state.

Malignancy

Malnutrition is common in patients with cancer, with as many as 70% suffering cancer cachexia. This is a condition characterised by severe weight loss, anorexia, a markedly decreased food intake, fatigue and a negative energy balance. Weight loss is the most significantly reported symptom and is linked to a poorer outcome in terms of response to treatment and survival. Nutrient intake is adversely affected in patients with cancer for a number of reasons. The side-effects of treatment may cause anorexia and vomiting. Some tumours release potent substances directly into the circulation that cause anorexia. In addition, psychological factors such as fear and anxiety in patients with cancer adversely affect appetite and food intake.

Nutritional intervention in patients with cancer improves nutritional indices in terms of body weight. However, whether nutritional interven-tion improves clinical outcome for the patient with cancer remains unclear. In spite of several studies, the outcome remains inconclusive.

Enteral tube feeding or PN may benefit those patients who are severely malnourished and those whose oral intake is to be severely restricted for some time, for example those undergoing GI surgery. For patients under-going bone marrow transplantation, PN or EN is implemented. The treat-ment regime for transplantation is protracted with long periods of a reduced oral intake and with some patients developing GI dysfunction. Artificial nutritional intervention in this group of patients is often required for survival, especially in children.

Parenteral nutrition should be used with caution in patients with end stage disease. This group of patients has been shown not to benefit from

PN; indeed, they have a paradoxically worsened prognosis secondary to the complications of parenteral feeding and the presence of a central venous catheter. Both initiating and withdrawing nutritional support in this instance is part of a controversial ethical debate, the decision involving the multidisciplinary team, the patient and his or her family.

A thorough bedside nutritional assessment is vital for the patient with cancer. Early referral to the dietitian for dietetic assessment and the introduction of snacks and high-calorie supplements may prevent the need for artificial nutritional intervention.

Acquired immune deficiency syndrome (AIDS)

This is a disease characterised by immune dysfunction secondary to the human immunodeficiency virus (HIV). At present there is no known cure for the disease and its progression is variable. There are few studies examining the effect of nutritional intervention upon the disease process. What is apparent is the frequent association of protein–energy malnutrition in patients with AIDS.

AIDS is a disease that causes wasting due to a number of factors. The disease may cause a mechanical dysfunction of the GI tract adversely affecting absorption of nutrients. There is a significant loss of appetite, frequent reports of diarrhoea and an increase in metabolic rate and energy expenditure. In addition, specific micronutrient deficiencies are reported, notably zinc, B complex vitamins, fat-soluble vitamins and the trace element selenium.

Early nutritional support is essential. Referral to a dietitian and the early institution of oral supplements is beneficial. If this proves to be insufficient to meet the nutritional needs, enteral feeding may be implemented. If long-term enteral tube feeding is required, a gastrostomy tube is preferable. However, nasogastric feeding is useful for the provision of short-term nutritional support, i.e. up to 1 month. If at all possible the enteral route is the preferred method of providing nutritional support for the patient with AIDS and is clinically effective in terms of repleting lean body tissues.

Parenteral nutrition is considered in the presence of GI tract dysfunction or when enteral feeding alone fails to meet the nutritional needs of the individual. There is some reluctance to commence parenteral feeding, however, owing to the recognised complication of catheter sepsis and the potential increased infection risk in patients with AIDS. This is an area requiring further research. Decisions to both commence and cease nutritional support may prove difficult ethical dilemmas. Such decisions are made in a multidisciplinary setting alongside the patient and family.

The patient with AIDS requires a full and detailed dietary and bedside nutritional assessment with introduction of early nutritional support. If EN or PN is required, feeding tubes and intravenous catheters are managed according to strict guidelines, reducing the risk of infection. Micronutrients are monitored and supplements administered as required.

Burns/sepsis/trauma

Patients with thermal injuries have unique nutritional demands due to the state of hypermetabolism that prevails following such injury. Energy and protein requirements are high in addition to the increased demand for fluid, electrolytes, vitamins and minerals. Careful evaluation is required as to the method of feeding and its composition.

Enteral feeding is the safest method of providing nutritional support in the patient with a thermal injury. Patients with less severe burns may maintain protein and energy balance with an oral supplemented diet. Patients with moderate to severe burns, however, may require enteral tube feeding, and this is commenced early in the post burn period. Despite the efficacy of enteral feeding in patients with thermal injury, it is not always tolerated. Patients with thermal injury may develop a paralytic ileus that prevents feeding directly into the GI tract. Sepsis also predisposes to the development of ileus. Patients with moderate to severe burns require frequent surgery for debridement and skin grafting, etc. This necessitates a preoperative 'starve' and the patient is deprived of nutrition for long periods of time. This is counteracted by the provision of PN that may be administered up to and during surgery. Parenteral nutrition is administered in the presence of GI tract dysfunction: paralytic ileus, pancreatitis and malabsorption. Parenteral nutrition is commenced 48–72 h post burn following adequate fluid resuscitation. It is often administered by the central route because of the increased risk of thrombophlebitis when using the peripheral route.

The maintenance of fluid and electrolyte homeostasis is vital in patients with burns. Similarly, the maintenance of an energy and nitrogen balance is crucial. Accurate fluid and electrolyte monitoring is essential, as is the monitoring of vitamins and trace elements. These are administered via the enteral or parenteral route in the thermally injured patient.

Patients who are critically ill, injured or septic all have increased nutritional requirements secondary to a hypermetabolic state. A nutritional assessment is performed early and repeated at intervals throughout the course of the injured patient's hospital stay. For those injured patients in whom nutrient intake is markedly reduced for a period of approximately 1 week, artificial nutritional support is not shown to alter outcome. For those patients in whom nutrient intake is reduced for a prolonged period, i.e. greater than 1 week, enteral or parenteral feeding is commenced. This prevents the onset of starvation and its associated complications.

Enteral feeding is implemented whenever possible owing to the reduced complication risks and the beneficial trophic effects upon GI tract mucosa. Significant benefits of EN over PN are seen in the most severely injured patients (ASPEN Board of Directors 1993). Some traumatic injuries, the onset of sepsis or multiorgan failure may render the GI tract dysfunctional and PN is implemented. In some patients with head injuries, gastric motility is delayed secondary to raised intracranial pressure, increasing the risk of pulmonary aspiration. The introduction of postpyloric feeding, for example feeding directly into the jejunum, may be considered to counteract this, although such feeding tubes are difficult to place and require frequent monitoring. Parenteral nutrition may be required for patients whose nutritional needs are unmet from enteral feeding alone. The transition from parenteral to enteral/oral feeding is made as soon as is possible.

Diseases in pregnancy

The administration of PN in pregnancy is rare. However, the advent of such a method of providing nutritional support has proved life-saving to some women and their unborn babies where nutritional state is compromised. Indications for PN include hyperemesis gravidarum (intractable nausea and vomiting) and diseases not associated with pregnancy, such as inflammatory bowel disease, bowel obstruction, cancer and pancreatitis.

An experienced support team is required to assess, monitor and evaluate the nutritional support, alongside an obstetrician to monitor maternal and foetal growth and development. If enteral tube feeding is tolerated, this is the preferred method of feeding. However, parenteral feeding has been shown to be safe and effective in terms of good clinical outcome for both the mother and the child (Kirby et al 1988).

PERIPHERAL PARENTERAL NUTRITION

Traditionally PN has been administered by the central route. This ensures the effective delivery of a large volume of hyperosmolar solution. Since the first description of a percutaneous approach to cannulation of the subclavian vein in the 1950s (Aubaniac 1952), line insertion has become a routine procedure, in some centres performed on the ward and increasingly by nurse practitioners. However, central venous cannulation is fraught with hazardous complications. These include insertion complications such as pneumothorax, and late onset mechanical complications such as line occlusion, thrombus formation and inadvertent removal. Central venous catheter sepsis is a well-cited complication that is known to reduce in the hands of an experienced operator (Mughal 1989).

Peripheral parenteral nutrition (PPN) is now considered to be 'the first choice for Total Parenteral Nutrition' (Payne-James & Khawaja 1993). It provides a safer and more cost-effective way to provide intravenous alimentation for the short term, i.e. 2 weeks. Consequently, it is not recommended in the following patients (Colagiavanni 1996):

- hypercatabolic/high energy demands
- high fluid demands
- long-term PN
- poor peripheral access
- chronic renal failure (due to risk of thrombosis in a vein required for dialysis).

The use of PPN is increasing. It is the most suitable method for administration of short-term parenteral nutrition, most courses of which are administered for less than 14 days (Payne James et al 1992). PPN is not without its complications, primarily the development of peripheral vein thrombophlebitis (PVT).

What is PVT?

There are many factors that cause PVT. It is characterised by erythema, pain and inflammation that occurs at the site of a peripheral line. It causes vein occlusion and extravasation of infusate into the surrounding tissues. There are histological changes that occur at the cannulation site:

sloughing of endothelial cells

↓

adherence of blood cells to the endothelial wall of the vein

↓

venous constriction

↓

release of inflammatory mediators

↓

thrombus formation

A simple and easy to use definition of PVT is the presence of two or more of the following signs:

- erythema
- pain
- swelling
- warmth
- palpable venous cord.

Two or more of the above signs would necessitate removal of the peripheral device and recannulation of another vein, preferably in the opposing limb.

Prevention of PVT

Many factors have now been identified that influence the development of PVT:

1. cannula size
2. material and length of cannula
3. osmolality and pH of the infusate
4. particulate matter
5. vein size and site of cannulation.

These are considered below (see also Box 3.6).

Cannula size

Small plastic cannulae are used in some centres for the administration of PPN. It is recommended that these cannulae remain in situ for 48 h after which they are removed and another inserted. This is time consuming for staff and has a low acceptability to patients enduring repeat cannulation every two days.

Studies have revealed lower incidence of PVT with finer bore catheters (Kohlhardt & Smith 1989, Madan et al 1992). Ultrafine catheters size 19–23 gauge are recommended. They are less imposing within a vein and create less trauma to the vein lining.

Material of cannula

The rigid nature of polyvinylchloride (PVC) cannulae is greatly linked to the formation of PVT. Polyurethane catheters have significantly less risk of PVT. The properties of polyurethane ensure a catheter that is soft and strong. In addition, polyurethane lessens the risk of thrombus formation by its ability to reduce adherence of platelets to its surface. These properties are also apparent with polyurethane central catheters.

Osmolality and pH of the infusate

This has tended to restrict the use of PPN. However, more recent studies

---

Box 3.6   Considerations to reduce PVT

- Use ultrafine e.g. 23 gauge catheters made from polyurethane
- Insert in a large vein away from a joint
- Atraumatic cannulation
- Use a 5 μm filter attached to the administration set
- Ensure osmolality of infusate is 800–1000 mosmol/L
- Ensure pH of infusate is 7.2–7.4

have shown that energy and protein requirements of patients on PN are less than previously thought. Patients rarely require more than 1500–2000 kcal and 10 g nitrogen unless hypermetabolic. Studies are variable although osmolalities of 800–1000 mosmol/L appear to be well tolerated (Payne-James & Khawaja 1993). Higher osmolalities have been reported (Kane et al 1996) that may increase the ability to feed patients with higher calories but in less volume. The pH of the infusate is recommended to be between 7.2 and 7.4. This is linked to a reduced incidence of PVT.

Lipid emulsions, carbohydrates and amino acids are administered by the peripheral route in all-in-one bags. The proportion of lipid as an energy source rarely exceeds 50%. Lipid has an additional property of protecting the endothelial wall of the vein.

Particulate matter

This forms part of a controversial debate as to the cause of line occlusion, thrombi and emboli in central and peripheral lines. The use of a 5 μm filter attached to the PN administration set filters large fat globules, precipitates, aggregates and solid particles. A 0.2 μm filter has the benefit of filtering bacteria but cannot be used when administering Intralipid® as the fat clogs the filter. The use of a filter has been shown to reduce significantly the incidence of PVT.

Vein size and site of cannulation

The site of cannulation is important. The vein should be large and cannulation is performed away from a joint. Trauma at the time of venepuncture reduces blood flow and increases the opportunity for the development of PVT. Cannulation sites for PPN are often the basilic and cephalic veins (Colagiavanni 1996) with insertion point above the antecubital fossa to prevent line disruption from movement at the elbow.

Nursing considerations

The peripheral line utilised for the administration of PPN is at risk of bacterial contamination. The key is prevention, and medical and nursing staff should adhere to strict guidelines of line management (Box 3.7). These

---

Box 3.7   Care of peripheral lines for PN

- Adequate handwashing and use of aseptic technique
- Regular observation of line site and maintenance of nursing documentation
- Flushing after discontinuation of infusion according to protocol
- Close liaison with NST/nurse

---

guidelines will alter according to individual trust/hospital. Strict hand-washing and an aseptic technique is utilised for peripheral cannulation and subsequent manipulations of the line. Prevention of complications is known to be enhanced with the instigation of a dedicated nutrition team and nutrition nurse, although the ward nurses are the best placed to detect the early signs of line sepsis.

The line should be regularly observed for the signs of PVT. The application of a transparent dressing at the site of insertion facilitates this.

The line is flushed following discontinuation of the infusion. Internal diameters of lumen are small and at risk of occlusion. Flushing of lines should be performed according to standard guidelines.

To prevent the venoconstriction and thrombus formation that inevitably occurs at the site of a peripheral line, glyceryl trinitrate patches (GTN) and topical non-steroidal anti-inflammatory agents (NSAID) may be used. The application of transdermal GTN patches has proved successful in pro-longing the survival of peripheral lines (Khawaja et al 1980). A 5 mg patch is applied daily to an area proximal to the site of the peripheral line. Side-effects include headaches. The severity of these is ameliorated by applica-tion of GTN patches on alternate days but relief of the headache should be obtained with the administration of simple analgesics, e.g. paracetamol.

The addition of heparin and hydrocortisone to the PPN solution is contro-versial. Heparin, an antithrombotic agent, has been shown to work effec-tively in the prevention of thrombus formation in fine peripheral lines. However, there is some concern over the effects of heparin on the stability of the parenteral solution with the formation of calcium–lipid–heparin complexes in all-in-one bags.

The advantages and disadvantages of PPN are summarised in Box 3.8.

SUMMARY

The ward nurse plays a vital role in the nutritional care of patients in hospital. A bedside nutritional assessment is a simple, yet effective, tool to recognise the patient at risk of or already suffering malnutrition.

Box 3.8   Advantages and disadvantages of PPN

Advantages
- Cost-effective
- Safe
- No X-ray required
- Lower risk of complications associated with central lines

Disadvantages
- Peripheral vein thrombophlebitis
- Not suitable for long-term PN

Assessment of GI function is essential to determine the method of nutritional support, whether this is parenteral or enteral.

Whenever possible, the enteral route is the preferred means of providing artificial nutritional support. However, in the presence of GI dysfunction, PN provides the energy, protein and micronutrients required for repletion of lean tissue and recovery. Parenteral nutrition is administered via the central or peripheral route, for long- or short-term support, respectively. Peripheral parenteral nutrition is administered successfully for up to a fortnight with a reduced incidence of PVT when following specific guidelines. The provision of optimal nutritional care to patients in hospital will not only reduce surgical complications, facilitate early recovery from illness and promote patients' physiological and psychological wellbeing, but will also ensure a more cost-effective service in healthcare.

REFERENCES

ASPEN (American Society for Parenteral and Enteral Nutrition) Board of Directors 1993 Special report: Guidelines for the use of nutritional support. Journal of Parenteral and Enteral Nutrition 17(4):1–52

Aubaniac R 1952 L'injection intravénouse sous claviculaire. Avantages et technique. Presse Médicale 60:1456

Colagiavanni L 1996 Peripheral benefits. Nursing Times 92(42):59–64

Eddington J, Kon P, Martyn CN 1997 Prevalence of malnutrition after major surgery. Journal of Human Nutrition and Dietetics 10:111–116

Hodder E 1873 Transfusion of milk in cholera. Practitioner 10:14–16

Kane KF, Colagiavanni L, McKiernan J et al 1996 High osmolality feedings do not increase the incidence of thrombophlebitis during peripheral IV nutrition. Journal of Parenteral and Enteral Nutrition 20(3):194–197

Khawaja HT, Campbell MJ, Weaver PC 1980 Effect of transdermal glyceral trinitrate on the survival of peripheral intravenous infusions: a double-blind prospective clinical study. British Journal of Surgery 67:311–312

Kirby DF, Fiorenza V, Craig RM 1988 Intravenous nutritional support during pregnancy. Journal of Parenteral and Enteral Nutrition 12:72–80

Klein S, Kinney J, Jeejeebhoy K et al 1997 Nutrition support in clinical practice: review of published data and recommendations for future research directions. Journal of Parenteral and Enteral Nutrition 21(3):133–150

Kohlhardt SR, Smith RC 1989 Fine bore silicone catheters for peripheral intravenous nutrition in adults. British Medical Journal 229:1380

Larsson J, Akerlind I, Permerth J, Hornqvist J 1995 Impact of nutritional state on quality of life in surgical patients. Nutrition 11(suppl 2):217–220

Lennard Jones JE 1992 A positive approach to nutrition as treatment. King's Fund Centre, London

McClave S, Greene LM, Snider H et al 1997 Comparison of the safety of early enteral vs parenteral nutrition in mild acute pancreatitis. Journal of Parenteral and Enteral Nutrition 21(1):14–20

McWhirter J, Pennington C 1994 Incidence and recognition of malnutrition in hospital. British Medical Journal 38:945–948

Madan M, Alexander DJ, Mcmahon MJ 1992 Influence of catheter type on the occurrence of thrombophlebitis. Lancet 339:101–103

Moy RJD, Smallman S, Booth IW 1990 Malnutrition in a UK children's hospital. Journal of Human Nutrition and Dietetics 3:93–100

Mughal MM 1989 Complications of intravenous feeding catheters. British Journal of Surgery 76:15–21

Norton B 1996 Nutritional assessment. Nursing Times 92(26):71–76

Payne-James J, de Gara CJ, Grimble GK et al 1992 Artificial nutrition support in hospitals in the United Kingdom – 1991: second national survey. Clinical Nutrition 11:187–192

Payne-James J, Khawaja H 1993 First choice for total parenteral nutrition: the peripheral route. Journal of Parenteral and Enteral Nutrition 17(5):468–478

Sitges-Serra A, Gil MJ, Rafecas A, Franch G, Jaurrieta E 1990 Nutritional issues in gastric cancer patients. Nutrition 6:171–173

Thomas TG 1878 The intra venous injection of milk as a substitute for the transfusion of blood. Illustrated by seven operations. New York Medical Journal 28:449–465

4

Choosing the appropriate catheter for patients requiring parenteral nutrition

Helen Hamilton

Introduction	Availability of suitable veins
Purpose and duration of therapy	Insertion of the central venous catheter
Clinical issues and potential	Available products
complications	Case studies
Patient considerations	Conclusion

INTRODUCTION

The successful provision of short- or long-term parenteral nutrition (PN) will depend on the selection of an appropriate catheter for the individual patient. The demands for blood sampling, short-term infusion, and intermittent long-term venous access for artificial nutrition are facilitated by the availability of sound and reliable central venous access. Owing to the ingenuity of recently developed materials and devices, modern central venous catheters (cvcs) are able to withstand conditions within the vascular system, thus reducing the risk of complications.

The choice of available devices suitable for the delivery of PN is vast. However, the objective of this chapter is not to recommend individual products, but rather to illustrate the importance of selecting the precise requirements of the device. The selection of an appropriate cvc may depend on numerous factors: venous availability, patient mobility, lifestyle, thrombosis, tumour, dominant preference, anatomical anomalies and the position in which the patient prefers to sleep. Often the nursing team, or in some cases the patient, will appreciate the difficulties that may present unless careful consideration is given to the selection of cvc and the proposed insertion site (see Box 4.1).

Reliable and appropriate venous access is essential to ensure the effective,

---

Box 4.1 Factors to be considered in selecting the venous access device

- Purpose and duration of therapy
- Clinical issues and potential complications
- Patient considerations
- Availability of suitable veins
- Method of insertion
- Expertise of operator
- Type of product available

---

safe delivery of PN. The increased use of ambulatory infusion pumps has demanded greater safety and reliability from intravenous access systems. Irrespective of complexity and cost, PN will be less than effective, and probably detrimental, when delivered via an inappropriately selected cvc.

PURPOSE AND DURATION OF THERAPY

The proposed duration of PN will often determine the type of venous access device to be used, and therefore the method by which it is to be inserted. Long-term PN therapy is usually administered using a cvc inserted using a percutaneous or internal jugular approach. Reliable, safe and simple venous access is essential for any type of intravenous therapy, but is particularly important if the patient will be assuming responsibility for the care of such a device.

PN administered over a brief period can often be achieved by either using a peripheral cannula or by gaining central venous access via a peripherally inserted central catheter (PICC), a relatively modern technique. In either method the access device can be removed promptly if enteral dietary intake becomes possible, patient stability is awaited, or phlebitis presents a problem. It is therefore worth considering the criteria for the appropriate selection of patients who may benefit from a PICC for PN. Most plastics used over a 48 h period via a peripheral approach will provide suitable access for PN. However, beyond this period peripheral administration of PN may cause phlebitis, resulting in pain, and may become cumbersome for the increasingly mobile patient. PN delivered by the peripheral route can be very successful for a brief period of time.

Historically, it is the nursing team who often consider the long-term implications of certain types of venous access, realising the limitations for their individual patients. Forward planning in the selection of the cvc and the demands required from the device will pay dividends, particularly in those patients who may have no peripheral access or who may require antibiotics and chemotherapy in addition to PN.

These factors must influence the type of device to be used, and whenever possible, discussion and explanation with the patient will result in a planned and structured approach to the safe delivery of PN.

CLINICAL ISSUES AND POTENTIAL COMPLICATIQNS

The clinical condition of the patient may often influence the method by which central venous access is to be gained. For example, a patient with pulmonary oedema may be unable to tolerate lying flat or head-down during the procedure. In this situation a peripheral approach to gaining central venous access may avoid distress to the patient and potential pneumothorax, which could be a complication if a percutaneous subclavian or internal jugular approach were used.

In Chapter 3 reference was made to the stability of the patient being essential prior to the insertion of a cvc. Unless stability can be achieved, a peripheral approach for the administration of nutritious agents may be more appropriate initially until such time as the patient's condition becomes more stable, when a tunnelled cvc may be more appropriate.

PATIENT CONSIDERATIONS

The selection of long-term venous access will often be successful if the patient is involved in the decision of which type of access device is to be used and, wherever possible, the site which is most acceptable. This requires careful patient preparation, as discussed in detail in Chapter 5.

A degree of patient compliance is necessary to guarantee a totally aseptic procedure, and the provision of PN much more likely to be successful if the patient is fully involved. Compliance can be encouraged by considering the factors relating to the individual patient that affect the selection and method of central venous cannulation (Box 4.2). For example, due to the clinical condition of the patient following surgery and possible discomfort, the prospect of adopting a head-down position while venous access is being attempted may not be conducive to all patients. Therefore, a procedure requiring less effort and discomfort may ensure patient compliance, yet still provide venous access for PN. In the event that PN is considered, a sensitive operator will take into account which side the patient sleeps, or may prefer the access device to be placed. The type of catheter material may also play a part in this factor as some plastics may kink more than others, causing the infusion pump to alarm if occlusion occurs. Sleep is a precious commodity in hospital!

The method of placement of the cvc can be a distressing prospect for many patients, particularly if they have had a previously unpleasant experience. Therefore, a sensitive and informed approach by the nursing team is vital in the preparation of the patient prior to the procedure. Informing the patient in advance of the procedure will often allay many preconceived ideas the patient may have. Personal experience suggests that it is helpful to discuss with the patient a résumé of the procedure, i.e. the level of

---

Box 4.2   Patient issues influencing the selection and method of central venous cannulation

- Patient compliance
- Body image
- Is needle phobia an issue?
- Will sedative agents compromise the patient's condition?

sedation, skin preparation, the introduction of local anaesthetic, the need for the operator to touch anatomical landmarks, plus the final application of sutures and dressings. The patient is then prepared for each stage of the procedure and will appreciate the importance of cooperation at the various stages. A creative and sensitive operator will ensure that the patient encounters the minimum of distress by discussing the siting options and potential problems that may occur when using short- or long-term venous access.

The issue of body image is an area that should not be overlooked in the selection of a cvc for PN. The prospect of a long-term venous access device positioned inappropriately may be demoralising not only for the patient, but also for partners and families. In children requiring PN, or prolonged periods of chemotherapy, it is not uncommon for the child to search the parent's chest for the detection of the parent's venous access device, particularly when anything other than a subcutaneous port is used.

AVAILABILITY OF SUITABLE VEINS

The venous network of any patient, in particular the patient requiring long-term PN or renal dialysis, is very precious. This issue is particularly pertinent in patients requiring recurrent central venous catheterisation for prolonged or repeated periods of home PN (HPN). In this instance central venous access becomes very difficult unless a structured approach to repeated cannulation is adopted, and the complications that may occur due to the material and size of the catheter considered.

Inevitably, the deciding factor when selecting a vascular device for the delivery of PN is the availability of a suitable vein (see Fig. 4.1). In many of the patients requiring this method of nutrition, previous hospital admissions involving PN, chemotherapy or antibiotic therapy may have resulted in what would have been ideal venous access becoming thrombosed or damaged, making future cannulation of the same vessel impossible. Anatomical anomalies such as tracheostomy or tumours involving the chest and neck may present difficulties for the operator planning to insert a cvc using the subclavian or jugular sites of access. It is therefore important to remember that an operator may be limited in the choice of venous access by the quality of the veins available. Hence, alternatives may have to be considered and influence the selection of the access device. For example, repeated percutaneous or surgical access to the subclavian vein may result in stenosis of the subcutaneous tissue and the vein wall, making the attempted insertion of a cannulation needle progressively more difficult.

Convenient and accessible central venous access is imperative for patients requiring HPN who will ultimately become responsible for the central

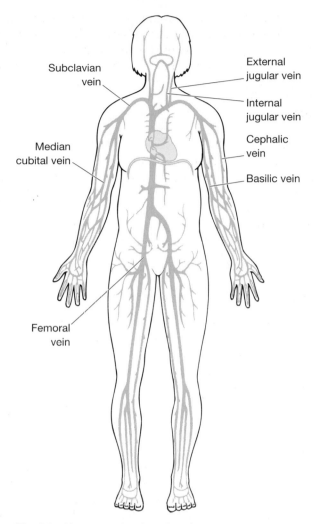

Fig. 4.1 Venous system insertion sites.

venous access device. Thus, a catheter placed directly into a neck vein would be entirely unsuitable. A more accessible site, for example the subclavian vein with the catheter tunnelled onto the chest wall, or a subcutaneous port, tunnelled and accessed via the chest or abdominal wall, may be more suitable. In selected cases a PICC via a peripheral arm vein situated in the antecubital fossa will ensure secure ease of access and confidence for the patient managing the catheter (see Fig. 4.2).

The advantages and disadvantages associated with the different veins used for PN are described below.

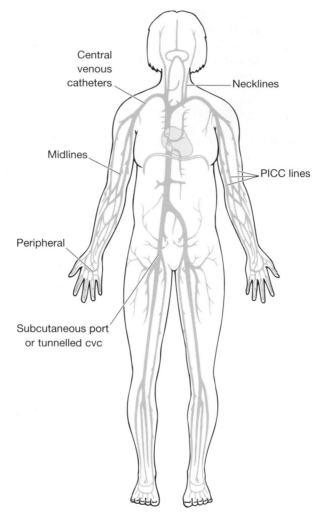

Fig. 4.2 Appropriate catheters and potential sites for parenteral nutrition.

Peripheral veins of the arm

The cephalic, basilic or median cubital veins of the forearm are often the first choice for the inexperienced operator who may wish to use the peripheral route for PN. Use of these veins will avoid the risk of major complications often associated with blind puncture of the great vessels of the neck and chest. The non-dominant arm should be used whenever possible.

In the very sick or compromised patient these veins may not be suitable due to inflammation from previous cannulation, thrombosis, or merely oedematous limbs, making attempted cannulation traumatic for the patient. Should this approach be the only possibility, an electronic Doppler device may be useful for the more experienced operator in identifying deep-seated vessels.

Proximal veins of the arm

The proximal veins of the arm are the axillary, proximal basilic and cephalic veins in the delto-pectoral groove. These veins are often larger than the previous group and can accommodate a longer-term indwelling cvc. Despite their size, these veins are more difficult to locate and are used infrequently as an alternative to the basilic, cephalic or forearm veins.

Subclavian vein

This vein is found under the clavicle and is approached using either a supraclavicular or infraclavicular approach. The subclavian vein is the most commonly used venous access for long-term PN, haemodialysis and chemotherapy, as the wide calibre of the vessel allows large volumes of fluid to be infused rapidly if necessary. A wide range of cvcs will be suitable for this approach, ranging from a fine-bore cvc to a larger device providing up to four lumens.

The added advantage of using the subclavian approach is that it allows the catheter to be secured to the chest wall, facilitated by a subcutaneous tunnel. Many of these catheters have a Dacron cuff which is positioned within the tunnel, which over a period of time will fibrose with the subcutaneous tissue within the tunnel, thus minimising movement and reducing the risk of infection.

Despite the popularity and convenience of using this route, serious and life-threatening complications may occur during insertion. It is for this reason that this approach should only be attempted by a skilled and experienced operator.

Internal jugular vein

This vein is situated in the neck and contained together with the carotid artery and vagus nerve in the carotid sheath. The internal jugular vein has become the accepted route for emergency venous access and major surgical cases. However, this is not a route recommended for the routine administration of PN, as the position of the catheter is uncomfortable for the patient. In addition, long-term nursing management of venous catheters placed in the neck is notoriously difficult. This site, despite having a low rate of complications related to insertion, has the highest infection rate of any insertion site, particularly when PN is used, owing to the complex and high glucose content of the nutritional regimen. Damage to the catheter in the suturing and securing stage of the procedure may cause extraluminal leakage of PN resulting in sudden and alarming swelling in the neck, which in a child may be fatal.

In a small group of patients where the subclavian vein is inaccessible, possibly due to tracheostomy, tumour or anatomical anomalies, the internal jugular vein may be used as venous access to the superior vena cava via a subcutaneous tunnel, and tunnelled onto the chest wall.

External jugular vein

This vein is usually superficial, clearly visible and easy to locate, making it an ideal vessel for emergency venous access and an inexperienced operator. Despite this reputation, the mobility of the vein may make it difficult to cannulate and it is only with flexible material used in the manufacturing process designed for this type of access that acute angles found in the external jugular vein can be negotiated. However, like the internal jugular vein, the external jugular vein is not suitable for PN because of the high risk of infection.

Following surgery, many patients return with venous access via the internal or external jugular vein with a dedicated lumen for the administration of PN. Administration of PN via this route is not recommended beyond 5–7 days owing to the high risk of infection and discomfort to the patient.

An experienced anaesthetist or vascular surgeon may, because of damage of the subclavian vein, cannulate the internal or external jugular vein and create a subcutaneous tunnel onto the chest wall, whereupon the cvc will be protected by the tunnel and infection will be avoided.

Femoral vein

This site of access will only be used for the delivery of PN when other available sites have either been exhausted or a clinical decision has been made to use the femoral vein (Fig. 4.3). The femoral vein is an important alternative to the subclavian route. Surgical intervention is the only method of insertion when selecting this site of access owing to the high risk of infection.

Complications associated with the femoral vein used for PN include infection and thrombosis. Significant research is being conducted into improving plastic materials suitable for this site. Silicone and silastic materials are the most commonly used in the femoral approach as these materials have the reputation of reduced thrombogenicity.

A high standard of management of the femoral site is required if infec-

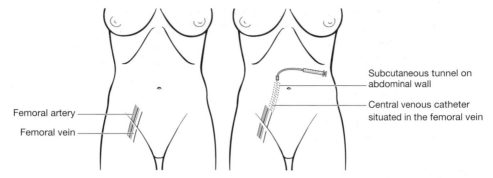

Subcutaneous tunnel on abdominal wall

Central venous catheter situated in the femoral vein

Femoral artery

Femoral vein

Fig. 4.3   Femoral venous access.

tion is to be avoided. Until the incisional wound has healed dressing can present a problem, and anal and skin hygiene is vital in limiting infection. In the majority of cases, a subcutaneous tunnel will be created on the abdominal wall to ensure that access to the vascular system is relocated, away from the groin area. Phlebitis, thrombosis and potential patient morbidity are well recognised in this type of venous access, which is why the femoral route will only be used in extreme and selected cases.

In the event that this route is to be used, thought should also be given to the patient's preferred position during sleep and other contributing factors, i.e. sporting activities such as shooting, archery, squash and sex, etc.

INSERTION OF THE CENTRAL VENOUS CATHETER

The ultimate decision as to which catheter and technique is to be used will depend on the following:

- expertise of the operator
- technique
- equipment available.

Expertise of the operator

The experience of the operator is a subject that is frequently discussed. This is an important consideration in a vascular procedure of this type, as there is the potential for damage to the patient. For this reason a simple and safe technique is more advisable than one that may result in serious complications. The necessary qualities for the operator selecting and inserting cvc for PN are listed in Box 4.3.

The success of any attempts at venous cannulation stems from the theoretical, practical knowledge and experience of the operator. However,

---

Box 4.3 Necessary qualities for the operator selecting and inserting cvcs for PN

- Expertise in technique
- Theoretical knowledge
- Practical experience
- Management and experience of complications associated with cvc insertion

---

despite most anaesthetists having considerable experience, with arm and neck veins in particular, no operator will be immediately familiar with all techniques and all the equipment available. It is therefore essential that an inexperienced operator selects an intrinsically safe procedure, despite a potentially lower success rate. Where a particular venous route is strongly indicated, the assistance of an experienced operator should always be sought for what is an invasive and often technically complex procedure.

Selection of a cvc is often made easier once the operator is defined. This will be made simpler if the operator's role is dedicated to the insertion of cvcs for the purpose of PN. The operator will become adept and confident in the chosen technique, thus reducing the risk of complications associated with central venous cannulation. Indeed, a dedicated operator has been shown to significantly reduce infection associated with the insertion of cvcs for PN (Hamilton 1995). However, this may not always be possible, and the choice of product may be limited to those suitable for the less experienced operator, encouraging a safer technique.

In either case, the choice of equipment and the method to be used should be used with due consideration of the patient's clinical condition and the anticipated duration of therapy.

Technique

An operator experienced in gaining central venous access will perform such a procedure using a structured approach, with consideration of the potential for future venous access. Centres providing a PN service often have a dedicated team of operators inserting cvcs for this purpose with a standard cvc and insertion method (Hamilton 1995). Technique considerations are highlighted in Box 4.4.

Box 4.4 Technique considerations for patients requiring central venous access for PN

- Operator's success and confidence in selected technique
- Surgical or percutaneous approach
- Suitability of technique in relation to patient's preference, age and clinical state
- Complication rate

The method employed to gain venous access for PN will often be determined by the operator's success in either the peripheral or central approach and the complications associated with both. The experience of the operator is therefore an important factor in the success and safety of the cannulation of veins to be used for PN.

Personal experience has demonstrated that success in central venous cannulation is increased when a cvc inserted for PN is made under elective circumstances. Detailed preparation is essential in order to ensure patient stability and thus reduce the risk of complications associated with the insertion of a cvc. In the event that the patient is unstable, an alternative method for providing PN using the peripheral route is always an option until such time as clinical stability is gained.

The basic equipment necessary to insert a cvc is a needle and a length of catheter. However, there are various methods by which the catheter will enter the vein. Cvcs inserted for PN are usually inserted using one of the following techniques:

- Seldinger wire approach via an introducer
- via a cannula
- surgically placed directly into the vein.

These are described briefly below, and in more detail in Chapter 6.

Seldinger wire approach

The usual method for the insertion of a tunnelled cvc is the Seldinger wire approach when the sites of access include the subclavian and jugular vessels. The Seldinger wire technique can also be used when inserting a PICC via an arm vein, although it will not always be possible to construct a subcutaneous tunnel.

Via a cannula

Access to the central venous system can also be gained by using a cannula over a needle, to aid in the cannulation of the vessels of the neck and chest. It is then possible to tunnel the catheter onto the chest wall, enabling ease of access in the management of the device. PICCs are usually inserted via a cannula or a needle, often with a Seldinger wire within the device to provide stiffness for insertion. The wire is removed when cannulation is achieved.

Surgical placement

Surgical placement of a cvc will require exposure of deep-seated vessels such as the femoral or cephalic veins. The selected vessel will be located, venotomy achieved, and the cvc will be introduced into the vascular system, whereupon a subcutaneous tunnel will be created either on the chest or abdominal wall.

PICC

Despite an apparent peripheral approach, the tip of a PICC is situated in the superior vena cava. This is achieved by the introduction of the catheter via the basilic vein. It is then advanced until the tip of the device is positioned in the superior vena cava. This provides an ideal alternative to the conventional method of gaining central venous access via the subclavian or internal jugular veins. The particular type of device shown in Fig. 4.4 has a three-way valve that opens and closes during negative or positive aspiration.

To ensure that the complications associated with this type of device are minimised, careful assessment by the operator is essential. The visibility and size of the vessels of the arm, clinical condition, patient mobility and comfort are all factors that must be considered prior to insertion of a PICC.

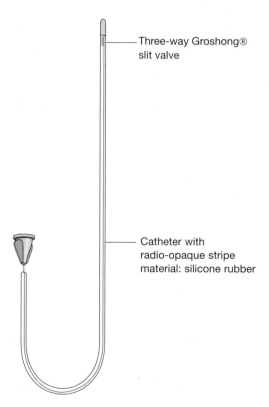

Three-way Groshong®
slit valve

Catheter with
radio-opaque stripe
material: silicone rubber

Fig. 4.4 Groshong® single-lumen PICC.

The size and visibility of the vein is a particularly important issue for the operator when considering the PICC for the administration of PN. Female patients often have smaller peripheral vessels and phlebitis may be caused by a PICC too large for the individual's vein, thus creating friction and pain.

Depending on the patient's clinical condition and haemodynamic state, the peripheral veins will vary in size and visibility. The common methods of encouraging dilation, such as the use of a tourniquet and the application of glyceryl trinitrate (GTN) patches, may be useful aids when attempting peripheral cannulation. However, care should be taken to monitor potential signs of phlebitis.

This method of gaining venous access can be a successful technique in the relatively inexperienced operator, providing a systematic and aseptic technique is adopted. PN administered via the peripheral route over long periods of time may not be ideal for all patients. Continuous infusion of PN may create restrictions and limit mobility. However, this type of device is ideal for bolus administration of certain therapies, and may even be suitable for overnight administration of PN in certain patients. PN is an ideal medium for multiplication of microorganisms, and so precise and aseptic management of this catheter is an essential aspect of patient care if infection is to be avoided. Box 4.5 summarises the issues that need to be considered when peripheral access is used for PN.

Equipment available

There are several factors that must be taken into account when considering what equipment to use (Box 4.6). Standardisation of a cvc will assist the users of a cvc to achieve competent management of a familiar vascular access device. The importance of a familiar product cannot be stressed more

---

Box 4.5   Considerations when peripheral access is to be used for PN

- Duration of PN
- Size, visibility and position of vessels
- Operator experience
- Patient mobility
- Patient comfort
- Management of device

Box 4.6   Factors to consider when selecting equipment

- Equipment
- Familiar product
- Availability
- Suitability of catheter material for individual patients
- Cost

strongly: it enhances the operator's experience in the selected technique of insertion, minimises waste and reduces complications associated with insertion. Confidence will be gained by the users of a familiar access device, rather than a variety, when differences in the management of these devices may increase the risk of confusion and complications.

Product availability may also influence the choice of device to be used, as well as the availability of compatible ancillary equipment necessary for repair purposes. Occasionally it may be necessary in the event of catheter damage to repair the access device. When selecting equipment to be used for long-term therapy, the facility to repair a cvc is essential and may prevent a patient requiring further venous access due to a damaged catheter. This is an avoidable complication.

When selecting a particular cvc consideration should be given to the merits of certain materials in the manufacture of the cvcs (see below) and the contraindications for use in certain groups of patients. Cost can also be minimised by standardising a product, thereby demonstrating a commitment that in turn may attract purchasing benefits from suppliers.

Nurse's role

As the knowledge base of nurses has expanded and extended roles developed, many responsibilities previously considered medical have been adopted by the nursing profession. Indeed, in a small number of centres throughout the UK, nurses are inserting intravenous access devices as part of their role, enhancing patient care, reducing infection and liaising with their nursing colleagues when selecting the appropriate type of cvc to be used in the delivery of PN, chemotherapy and antibiotics.

AVAILABLE PRODUCTS

As mentioned above, when choosing the cvc consideration must be given to the material, as well as factors such as size, length, and whether the catheter should have a single or multiple lumens.

Catheter materials

When central or peripheral administration of PN is to be considered, the performance and success of any cvc will depend on certain properties in the design, for example flexibility, thromboresistance, resistance to kinking, and cost. When considering catheter material the characteristics of each type should be addressed. The stiffness of some catheters may cause severe damage to the vein wall and may also facilitate thrombosis as a result of pressure to the wall of the vein. In principle, the ideal catheter material for long-term central venous access will be chemically inert, nonthrombogenic, flexible and radio-opaque. However, this is a tall order even for modern-day plastics.

The most commonly used polymers, or plastics, found in the manufacture of vascular devices include: polyurethane, silicone, polyvinylchloride (PVC), fluoropolymer (Teflon), polyethylene and elastomeric hydrogel. The advantages and disadvantages of these plastics are discussed in Table 4.1.

Polyurethane is a plastic that currently enjoys popularity owing to its superior strength over the softer, more pliable materials. In addition, this material has shown resistance to wearing over prolonged periods, it will recover its shape after deformation, and it is resistant to heat degradation. These qualities aid the operator as they can reduce the risk of kinking, deformation and external occlusion.

Silicone is a sophisticated and versatile material used in the manufacture of specialised long-term central venous devices. Silicone avoids the short-comings of simpler catheter materials, which can include infection, phlebitis and catheter-related pain. Silicone is also regarded as the least traumatic and thrombogenic material of the materials used in the manufacture of modern cvcs.

Table 4.1 Properties of catheter materials

Material	Advantages	Disadvantages
Polyurethane	Strong Kink-resistant qualities Thromboresistant Compatible with infusional agents Softens within the body Percutaneous insertion possible Small lumen size possible	Can kink
Silicone	Compatible with most infusional agents Thromboresistant Soft, pliant and comfortable for patient Tolerant of chemicals Percutaneous placement possible Low surface energy Large lumen size possible	Poor tolerance to pressure May knot
PVC	Softens within body	High absorption of certain drugs High incidence of thrombosis
Teflon	Resistant to chemicals Low surface energy Slippery	Kinks readily Increased risk of thrombosis Stiff
Polyethylene	Strong Permeable to O_2 and CO_2 Resistant to chemicals, fat and oil	Stiff Kinks Small lumens
Elastomeric hydrogel	Softens within the body	Size of catheter changes on fluid contact

Teflon was popular some years ago in the manufacture of peripheral cannulae. However, with the advanced and superior strength of polyurethane, this material is now rarely used.

The risk of thrombus formation while using a cvc for whatever type of treatment is one which can be significantly reduced if the catheter material is considered with care and the catheter maintenance protocol adhered to. A comparison of polyurethane and silicone would certainly suggest that the stiffer polyurethane more readily facilitates the formation of thrombus, making the softer and more pliable silicone the preferable material to use for a cvc (Linder et al 1984).

Studies in the thrombogenicity of varying materials indicate that the actual chemical composition may be an important factor in the incidence of thrombophlebitis (Borow & Crowley 1985). Many experiments using heparin coating and bonding of cvcs have been disappointing and have provided little evidence to suggest that thrombogenicity is reduced in comparison with plain and uncoated catheters.

In essence, despite modern developments in the field of cvcs, it would appear that although the chemical composition of the catheter material is an important factor when considering the thrombogenic risks associated with central venous access, the size and stiffness of each individual device must be given careful consideration.

Catheter size

In the administration of PN it is generally recommended that the largest catheter should be used in relation to the patient's size and planned duration of PN. This is of particular importance for patients requiring HPN, when a build-up of fibrin and lipid deposits within the catheter lumen may produce an occlusion.

Single or multiple lumens?

The question of the number of lumens required should also be addressed at this stage. Due to the small lumen size of double-lumen PICCs, these catheters may not be suitable for long-term PN.

Ideally a single-lumen, dedicated cvc is probably the approach least likely to result in complications associated with blockage and infection. However, few acutely ill patients will require purely PN with no other intravenous therapies.

Multilumen catheters may be essential in patients requiring bone marrow transplantation or other therapy, in which case the dedication of one lumen for PN will ensure the minimisation of contamination. This will only be guaranteed if the same respect of aseptic technique is afforded to all the lumens of the catheter.

Length

Length is an important measurement in any catheter used for PN. Many centres recommend accurate documentation of the catheter length, particularly when PICCs are used, plus the length from skin exit to Luer connection (Gabriel 1996). This is a particularly useful observation should an uncuffed catheter be used, which may at some time become displaced, whereupon PN could infuse into extravascular tissue.

CASE STUDIES

The following Case Studies illustrate the relevance of appropriate patient-focused catheter selection.

Case Study 4.1

Mrs Jones, a 56-year-old lady weighing 50 kg, was admitted under the care of the general surgeons complaining of abdominal pain. Her only previous medical history was severe stress-related asthma. Following examination and abdominal X-rays a diagnosis of abdominal sepsis, due to a possible peritoneal abscess, was made. Mrs Jones was observed and administered intravenous fluids via a peripheral cannula in her hand. A nasogastric tube was inserted to relieve her symptoms of nausea and vomiting.

On admission Mrs Jones' biochemistry was normal apart from a low serum albumin. Haematology revealed a slightly low haemoglobin and elevated white blood count (wbc). After 2 days Mrs Jones continued to vomit despite the presence of the nasogastric tube. A diagnosis of small bowel obstruction was made and, in view of her history of a week without nutrition, falling weight, low serum albumin plus the uncertainty of the duration of her obstruction, the decision was made to provide Mrs Jones with artificial, intravenous nutrition to reduce the risk of malnutrition. With the provision of PN it would also be possible to include antigastric erosion agents to the PN, thus avoiding the potential development of stress-related ulcers. At this point there were no plans to operate on Mrs Jones and therefore, in order to deliver PN, a cvc had to be placed.

Prior to the procedure, preliminary considerations were taken into account:

- Blood was taken to establish safe parameters of haematology and in particular coagulopathy, a routine assessment necessary prior to the insertion of any cvc.
- Discussion and explanation to Mrs Jones of the proposed form of nutrition, and the method of delivery.
- Informed patient consent, with Mrs Jones being made aware of the potential complications that can occur during the insertion of a cvc.
- Assessment by the operator of Mrs Jones' available venous access.

Mrs Jones was examined by the operator and found to have satisfactory peripheral veins in the antecubital fossa. Her skin condition appeared reasonable, if somewhat dry. The full procedure was discussed with the patient. The merits of the proposed access device and the complications that might occur during the insertion and during the delivery of PN were explained clearly to Mrs Jones by the operator. Mrs Jones was experiencing persistent nausea, which was unrelieved by antiemetic therapy. In view of this it was felt, following discussion with the patient, medical and nursing teams, that a peripherally inserted cvc (PICC) would be the most appropriate method of delivering short-term PN to this patient. This type of device would avoid the patient being placed in the Trendelenburg position (see Fig. 5.1) and, in view of the probable

Case Study 4.1   (*contd*)

short duration of PN, plus the absence of multiresistant *Staphylococcus aureus* (MRSA), a dedicated PICC, peripheral cannula or mid-line catheter would be ideal.

Although intravenous antibiotics were considered by the medical team to be a strong possibility for Mrs Jones, because of her unresolved abdominal sepsis, it was felt that her peripheral vessels would provide adequate access if this became necessary. This was also supported by the patient. Mrs Jones was relieved to understand that little effort was required by her during the insertion procedure.

On receipt of normal haematology results, informed patient consent and detailed discussion with the proposed nursing users of the PICC, the patient was prepared for the insertion. In order that a painless insertion could take place a local anaesthetic agent was applied to Mrs Jones' right arm in the area of the antecubital fossa (Wig & Johl 1990). Approximately 1 h later, once the local anaesthetic agent had taken effect, the insertion procedure could begin. As Mrs Jones was nursed in a side room it was considered a sufficiently clean area for this procedure, with the added advantage of few interruptions.

Mrs Jones was requested to extend her right arm at a 45° angle from her chest and place her arm comfortably, supported by a pillow, on a bed table. An approximate measurement was made from Mrs Jones' antecubital fossa to the shoulder to mid-sternal notch, providing the operator with the necessary information to site the catheter accurately in its final position in the superior vena cava (svc), the recommended position for a PICC (Gabriel 1996). Using this method of measurement for Mrs Jones resulted in a length of 54 cm.

A tourniquet was applied to Mrs Jones' right upper arm to encourage engorgement of the selected vessel. The selected insertion area was cleansed thoroughly and aseptically with an antiseptic solution by the operator, who wore sterile, unpowdered gloves, as a precaution taken to avoid phlebitis. (Maki et al (1991) have published extensive research regarding effective skin preparation, indicating that chlorhexidine 2% is the most effective cleansing solution, if allowed to dry.)

Mrs Jones' arm was draped in sterile towels. A 16 gauge cannula was inserted into the basilic vein. This vein is often considered to have a more direct route to the great vessels of the chest, with fewer junctions for the advancing catheter to negotiate. Using the catheter through the needle approach, a 4FG, 60 cm PICC was introduced into the cannula and advanced approximately 10 cm through the cannula, whereupon the tourniquet was released.

Mrs Jones was requested to turn her head to her right and place her chin on her chest, aiding and preventing the advancement of the catheter into the veins of the neck. The remaining length of the catheter was gently advanced until the tip of the catheter was considered to be in the svc. Approximately 6 cm of the catheter remained exposed on the patient's arm.

Following insertion the PICC was aspirated with a 10 ml syringe to ensure venous position. It was flushed with 10 ml of 0.9% sodium chloride followed by 5 ml of heparinised saline 10 units per ml. A 10 ml syringe is the smallest syringe recommended for this type of catheter because of the high pressure generated by a smaller syringe and possible perforation of the PICC as a result of this pressure (Gabriel 1996).

The PICC entry site was cleaned and secured using steristrips. A small non-adherent dressing was applied and covered with a transparent and waterproof dressing. Below this dressing an additional securing mechanism was applied to Mrs Jones' forearm, using an adhesive pad to which the catheter was fixed and which restricted movement of the PICC catheter (Fig. 4.5). The site was finally covered with an elasticated bandage to ensure that the PICC did not get caught on equipment and clothing. Mrs Jones was relieved the procedure had been so swift with no experience of discomfort during the insertion of the PICC catheter.

A chest X-ray was performed, which confirmed the correct position of the PICC. The recommended position for a cvc for the delivery of PN is the junction between

Case Study 4.1   (*contd*)

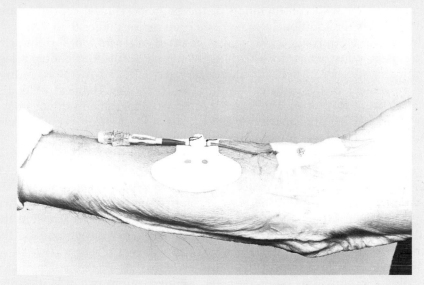

Fig. 4.5   PICC inserted in a patient.

the superior vena cava and the right atrium (RA). The nursing team and patient were informed of the correct position by the operator. Mrs Jones' PN was commenced that night, administered via an infusion pump.

The ward nursing team checked the dressing site the following day, using a two-person technique in case the catheter was dislodged during the redressing process. Biochemistry and haematology blood samples were obtained from Mrs Jones' peripheral veins twice a week with no difficulty or distress to her. Within a week Mrs Jones' bowel obstruction began to resolve and she was able to tolerate clear fluids and progress to a light diet. Once enteral feeding was clearly established PN was reduced and finally stopped.

On cessation of artificial nutrition, the PICC was removed by pulling the catheter gently from the vein. The tip was sent for microbiology, culture and sensitivity. Mrs Jones went home 3 days later enjoying a normal light diet and continued to make a full recovery.

The issues considered in Case Study 4.1 are summarised in Box 4.7.

Box 4.7   Summary of Case Study 4.1

- Good patient selection
- Patient assessment
- Patient compliance
- Team and patient involvement in decision-making
- Short-term PN
- Patient-related stress factors considered
- Asthmatic patient, unsuitable for a subclavian approach owing to the increased risk of pneumothorax.
- Alternative venous access for other therapies

The selection of such a dedicated device for Mrs Jones and her requirement for short-term PN was successful due to careful patient assessment, together with consideration of the patient's clinical condition and requirements for additional intravenous preparations other than PN.

In this Case Study the catheter was inserted into Mrs Jones' right arm. If possible, when using a PICC, it is preferable to use the patient's less dominant side, which will inevitably be used less and therefore reduce the movement of the catheter, limiting the risk of mechanical phlebitis. In addition, it is important to attempt to ensure that patients always have one arm free of infusions. With both arms restricted, movement, even attempting to take a sip of water, becomes impossible!

Care was taken to position the catheter correctly, by taking a measurement of the distance from the antecubital fossa to the shoulder to midsternal notch, which in Mrs Jones' case was 54 cm. Each patient will obviously vary in size and therefore measurement becomes an individual issue. The measurement of each patient will influence to what extent the catheter is advanced into the vein and the length remaining outside the patient.

In this Case Study the peripheral and proximal veins were adequate for peripheral cannulae to be used in the administration of antibiotics and blood sampling. Additional lumens for the administration of other agents were therefore unnecessary. Wherever possible, a dedicated catheter purely for the administration of PN is highly recommended and will reduce the risk of catheter-related sepsis.

Although in this case a PICC was selected, a mid-arm catheter, inserted in a similar way, but situated in the cephalic or basilic vein, short of the svc, would also have been suitable. Placement of a true peripheral cannula might not have been successful due to the nature of Mrs Jones' symptoms and frequent movement when vomiting, making venous access somewhat unstable and increasing the risk of mechanical phlebitis.

Case Study 4.2

Mr Lee, a 30-year-old married gamekeeper, was admitted for the eighth time in the past 4 years, suffering from recurrence of Crohn's disease. He was admitted to the Gastroenterology Department for investigations and assessment of his disease.

On examination Mr Lee appeared gaunt, obviously having lost a considerable amount of weight, lethargic and demoralised. He reported having had considerable time away from work owing to his lack of energy, and the frequency of bowel actions were causing him embarrassment at work to the extent that he felt he could no longer work. In addition, his wife of 1 year was finding it difficult to accept his condition. The husband she married was a fit, active and sporty individual with much energy who enjoyed socialising. Now, after such a brief period, Mr Lee was exhausted, demoralised and merely wanted to sleep.

On admission to the ward investigations were commenced. Blood tests revealed that Mr Lee had a markedly elevated C-reactive protein (CRP), a low haemoglobin,

Case Study 4.2   (*contd*)

low albumin and deranged trace elements and vitamins. Small bowel studies revealed extensive Crohn's disease with the addition of a small bowel fistula in the ileum. A drain was inserted to aid drainage of this and the decision to commence PN was made. His enteral dietary intake was stopped.

On examination it was apparent that Mr Lee had lost a considerable amount of weight with both upper arms noticeably wasted. Numerous scars on either side of his chest below the clavicle suggested previous subclavian approaches for PN. Grossly dilated and visible veins appearing only on the right side of his chest was another observation made by the nursing staff.

Mr and Mrs Lee were informed of the decision to use artificial methods in the provision of nutrition. Mr Lee had in fact received PN many times before at another hospital and, although recalling how rapidly his nutritional state had improved, he had not received PN during his relationship with his wife. Mr Lee was naturally apprehensive at her reaction to a venous access device, particularly as on this occasion it would appear the duration of PN might stretch to months rather than the days he had experienced previously. Mrs Lee understood the importance of ensuring her husband gained urgent nourishment from PN, but was unprepared for the proposed duration.

The benefit of a team approach in the forward planning of Mr Lee's care was both demanding and yet challenging. In order to enable him to return to his previous state of mind and health, the delivery of PN was paramount to his future. Considerable time in counselling was necessary to educate both Mr and Mrs Lee to the potential merits and difficulties associated with this type of nutrition. With all the information available to them Mr and Mrs Lee decided to take the advice of the medical team and learn the skills involved in the administration of PN in their home while the fistula healed, rather than for Mr Lee to remain in hospital for a prolonged period.

The question of venous access to achieve this end was a demanding selection as Mr Lee obviously wished to return to his sporting activities and his job. As a gamekeeper he was required to arrange shoots for his farmer employer and maintain a selection of pheasants for the shoots in addition to other physical responsibilities around the farm. As a newly married man body image was obviously an important issue. Mr Lee's sporting activities included scuba diving and an occasional game of fairly competitive squash, although neither of these activities would be an immediate option until his poor nutritional state had been addressed.

The question of suitable available venous access devices was discussed at length with both Mr and Mrs Lee. Two devices were considered: the Port-a-Cath® and the double-lumen silicone catheter.

The Port-a-Cath is a titanium reservoir that is placed surgically in a subcutaneous pocket on the chest wall, abdominal wall or on the forearm (Fig. 4.6). The subclavian or cephalic veins are often the first choice of access and the catheter is inserted into the vein and attached to the reservoir. The patient may then access the silicone diaphragm of the reservoir via the skin, which over time becomes desensitised to frequent puncture. The femoral vein may also be used as a source of access in this method of providing a long-term venous access, by creating a subcutaneous pocket to house the device in a position that is agreed by the patient. The basilic or cephalic veins may also be used, with the implantable port positioned on the forearm. With any of these types of devices a strict sterile surgical placement is necessary, given the exposure of the subclavian vein and creation of the subcutaneous pocket to house the venous access port.

The second device for Mr Lee to consider was a double-lumen silicone catheter that would exit at nipple level, below a subcutaneous tunnel. This type of device could be placed percutaneously, without the need for general anaesthetic, on the ward in familiar surroundings with familiar staff.

After considerable thought and discussion with other patients who had experience with both types of device, Mr Lee decided to opt for a Port-a-Cath, which would provide the best venous access device and permit a relatively normal routine, given

Case Study 4.2 (*contd*)

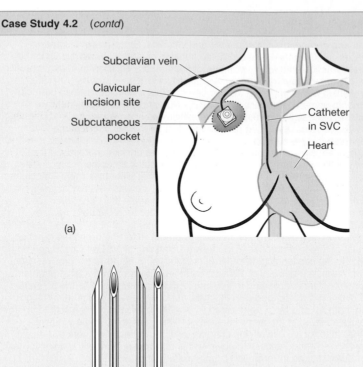

Subclavian vein

Clavicular
incision site

Subcutaneous
pocket

Catheter
in SVC

Heart

(a)

(b) Huber Regular

Fig. 4.6 (a) Subcutaneous port with subcutaneously implanted reservoir. (b) Needles used to access a Port-a Cath.

the unusual circumstances of his lifestyle. Mr Lee was made aware of the potential difficulties the operator may experience in the location of an appropriate vessel due to previous cannulation attempts from previous episodes of PN.

Mr Lee's dominant side was documented and the preferred site marked. He was reassured that if at all possible the Port-a-Cath would be sited on the selected side in a position that would not create difficulties for him at work.

Prior to the procedure, the following considerations were taken into account:

- Informed consent was obtained.
- Blood was taken for full blood count, coagulopathy, i.e. prothrombin time (PT) and activated partial thromboplastin time (APPT), to ensure these factors were within the normal parameters.
- In view of previous episodes of PN, plus the dilated, unilateral dilated vessels observed on Mr Lee's chest suggesting thrombosis may exist, venography was arranged to assess the patency of the great vessels of the chest.
- Assessment of allergic status regarding dressing to be used was carried out.

Case Study 4.2   (*contd*)

- The patient was made fully aware of the potential initial discomfort of a newly placed Port-a-Cath. Often the specially designed needle, a Gripper or Huber needle, which gains access to the silicone reservoir, will be inserted during the procedure by the surgeon, to alleviate some discomfort immediately post operatively.
- Previous anaesthetic experiences were assessed by the anaesthetic team.
- Proposed venous access sited by marking Mr Lee's chest, ensuring that he agreed with the site and was able to reach or physically see the site in question.
- The specific and correct device was ordered and made available for theatre on the planned day of insertion. Because of the high cost of this type of device, i.e. >£500, it is common for the device to be ordered for the individual patient.

Mr and Mrs Lee awaited the insertion of the device with some degree of trepidation, but were satisfied that every alternative had been explored. On return from theatre the Port-a-Cath site was checked and found to be oozing. An extension set, with the Gripper or Huber needle, was in position in order to avoid the necessity of needle puncture over a sensitive wound site.

The area was redressed using a non-adherent dressing covered with a transparent waterproof dressing until the incision had healed and the sutures removed. This normally takes approximately 7–10 days and during this period it is of great importance that the suture line remains dry, thus encouraging a cosmetic and aesthetic scar.

Over a period of time the area of skin above the silicone reservoir will become desensitised and less painful when the Huber access needle punctures the skin. Initially, Mr Lee applied a local anaesthetic agent over the site for an hour prior to reduce any discomfort when commencing PN via the Port-a-Cath.

Mr and Mrs Lee were delighted with the appearance of the incision housing the device and appreciated the consideration that had been afforded in the decision-making process of device selection.

The issues considered in Case Study 4.2 are summarised in Box 4.8.

Box 4.8   Summary of Case Study 4.2

- Detailed patient examination and assessment
- Appropriate venous access device selected following detailed discussion and consideration of the patient's lifestyle
- Careful assessment of vascular patency in view of previous episodes of PN and unilateral presentation of dilated collateral blood supply to chest
- Assessment of whether patient, in view of his dislike of needles, would tolerate daily puncture of his skin when commencing administration of PN
- Counselling and discussion with patient and wife to ensure both parties were informed and thus able to make the decision as to which device was most suitable
- The importance of body image in a newly married couple

Case Study 4.3

Mrs Dodd, a 45-year-old lady with Crohn's disease, was admitted from home complaining of 'leakage' of a foul-smelling liquid from an area on her abdominal wall. Investigations included a small bowel enema which demonstrated an enterocutaneous fistula originating in the ileum, which was leaking small bowel contents onto the surface of her skin. This was causing great distress to the patient, not only because she was very aware of the odour emitted from the site, but also due to the excoriation caused to her skin.

In addition to her discomfort, Mrs Dodd's peripheral venous access was poor and she was distraught at the thought of regular painful attempts to obtain blood samples. Unfortunately Mrs Dodd had experienced similar symptoms 2 years previously, resulting in a period of PN at home. Mrs Dodd had successfully administered this over a 6 month period herself, following tuition from the nursing team at her local hospital, while awaiting the fistula to heal.

On this occasion a single-lumen Hickman-type catheter had been inserted and, although satisfactory in terms of providing an administration route for PN, it was not considered appropriate to harvest blood from the catheter due to the risk of infection, potential occlusion caused by a build-up of blood agents within the catheter, together with fat deposits from the PN.

Mrs Dodd was referred to the PN and stomatherapy teams for the management of her small bowel fistula. Following discussion with the patient, the medical team and the specialist teams, it was agreed with the patient and family to attempt to heal the fistula conservatively by providing PN. This would hopefully avoid exacerbation of her symptoms of small bowel content leakage via the fistula if enteral nutrition was continued. A very small amount of enteral supplementation was recommended to preserve gut integrity and prevent bacterial translocation (Alexander 1998).

The stomatherapy team were instrumental in ensuring that the painful site on Mrs Dodd's abdomen was dry and that the small bowel contents drained into an odour-free drainage appliance system, attached to the patient. Mrs Dodd elected a percutaneous method of central venous insertion. Physical examination and assessment, haematology assessment and coagulopathy to ensure clotting studies were within normal limits were carried out, and informed consent was obtained.

Mrs Dodd, having received PN before, was reminded of the forthcoming procedure by the operator and the nursing team, and the potential complications of insertion were also explained. The patient was reassured and reminded that in the hands of an experienced operator these complications were far less likely to occur, but legally, potential complications must be discussed with the patient.

The insertion site and final position of the device were also discussed between patient and operator. Unfortunately, the potential for repeated episodes of PN in Mrs Dodd's case were fairly high, and therefore planning for future central venous catheterisation was not only cosmetically important for the patient but a systematic approach to the placement of the cvc would reduce the risk of complex and traumatic cvc placements in the future. (Alternating the site of cannulation, commencing at a lateral point and maintaining a more medial access on each new course of PN will ensure that virgin or less traumatised tissue will be available for access in the future delivery of PN.)

Following discussion with the patient it was decided to insert a tunnelled 9FG double-lumen silicone cvc to enable one lumen to be used for PN and the other lumen to be used for blood sampling, in view of Mrs Dodd's poor peripheral access and her dread of repeated venepuncture (Fig. 4.7). Regular blood sampling would be necessary for monitoring electrolyte balance associated with her enterocutaneous fluid losses and monitoring of PN.

The cvc was inserted percutaneously using a benzodiazepine agent as a method of sedation. Mrs Dodd, although lightly sedated, had no memory of the procedure and was relaxed and cooperative throughout.

Case Study 4.3 *(contd)*

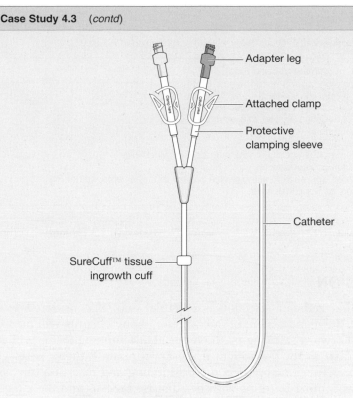

Adapter leg

Attached clamp

Protective
clamping sleeve

Catheter

SureCuff™ tissue
ingrowth cuff

Fig. 4.7 Double-lumen cuffed catheter.

During the next 4 months the double-lumen catheter performed admirably, with no difficulties experienced by the patient. Her relief at blood sampling via the catheter each week, rather than venepuncture, was very apparent, and Mrs Dodd took fastidious care of the flushing technique recommended in her maintenance protocol. At no time did she experience occlusion difficulties and always used the larger lumen for the administration of PN, ensuring the infusion was completed prior to blood sampling from the smaller lumen.

When not in use, Mrs Dodd coiled the catheter either in her bra, which was invisible when wearing clothes, even low-cut summer attire, or contained the catheter in a cotton pouch which she pinned to her blouse when not wearing her bra. Mrs Dodd fortunately did not enjoy swimming – this sport is not advised in patients with fistulae or this type of venous access, and in particular in those patients who may be immunosuppressed due to their therapies, as there is a real risk of infection associated with swimming.

Six months later, once her fistula had healed, her cvc was removed surgically using a local anaesthetic agent. In the hands of a sensitive and experienced operator, the scar caused by the removal of the fibrosed Dacron cuff situated in the subcutaneous tissue under the skin was minuscule, with little scarring.

Mrs Dodd was discharged and an appointment made for her to attend the outpatient clinic where she was seen by her gastroenterologist and dietitian. At this time her enteral nutritional intake, weight and general assessment would ensure the issues relating to her fistula had finally resolved.

Case Study 4.3   (*contd*)

The issues considered in Case Study 4.3 are summarised in Box 4.9.

Box 4.9   Summary of Case Study 4.3

- Good patient assessment
- Patient's competence in aseptic technique
- Level of sedation agreed with patient
- Needle phobia
- Regular blood sampling
- Familiar venous access device made selection simple
- Use of lumens considered
- Structured approach to siting device in view of further episodes of PN
- Scarring issues considered

CONCLUSION

Care regarding catheter selection is essential and, if considered by all concerned in the management of the catheter, many benefits will manifest themselves. Forward thinking by the medical and nursing teams will alleviate much distress for the patient if the appropriate catheter is selected initially. Successful catheter selection, positioning and insertion can assist the patient in coming to terms with her disease process and the effective methods by which this can be treated.

Using assessment to aid in the appropriate selection of a venous access device will provide our patients with the confidence to know they have the best possible device for their therapy and lifestyle.

REFERENCES

Alexander JW 1998 Procedures of Nutritional Society 57(3): 389–393
Borow M, Crowley J 1985 Evaluation of central venous catheter thrombogenicity. Acta Anaesthesiologia Scandinavica 81 (suppl):59
Gabriel J 1996 Peripherally inserted central catheters: expanding UK nurses' practice. Surgical Nurse 5(2):71–74
Hamilton H 1995 An extended role. Nursing Times
Linder L, Curelaru I, Gustavsson B et al 1984 Material thrombogenicity in central venous catheterisation: a comparison between soft, antebrachial catheters of silicone elastomer and polyurethane. Journal of Parenteral and Enteral Nutrition 8:399
Maki D, Ringer M, Alvardo C 1991 Prospective randomised trial of povidone iodine, alcohol and chlorhexidine for prevention of infection with central venous and arterial catheters. Lancet 383:339–343
Wig J, Johl K 1990 Our experience with Emla cream (for painless venous cannulation in children). Indian Journal of Pharmacology 34(2):130–132

FURTHER READING

Andrews J 1995 Chronic venous access: the role of interventional radiology. Paper presented at 9th National Association of Vascular Access Networks (NAVAN) Conference, September 1995, Salt Lake City, Utah

Goodwin M, Carlson I 1993 The peripherally inserted catheter: a retrospective look at 3 years of insertions. Journal of Intravenous Nursing 16(2):92–103

5

Preparing the patient for central venous catheter insertion

Helen Balsdon

Introduction	Practical requirements
Aims of patient preparation	Helpful hints in pre-catheter insertion
Provision of information	Conclusion
Patient concerns	

INTRODUCTION

This chapter will initially discuss the provision of information regarding insertion of a central venous catheter (cvc) and will lead on to practical indicators regarding the preparation of the patient. Nurses using cvcs should have some knowledge of how to prepare patients for a cvc, and an understanding of why good preparation is so important.

Although this book focuses upon parenteral nutrition (PN), there are a variety of other indications for cvc insertion, such as bone marrow transplantation, long-term antibiotic or drug therapy, or long-term blood product support. As a result of this, the patient may be based on any ward within the acute hospital setting, including medical, surgical, or speciality settings such as gastroenterology, renal and haematology. This chapter will look at pre-catheter insertion, and will be of use to all nurses who have to prepare a patient for placement of a central venous catheter.

AIMS OF PATIENT PREPARATION

Placement of a catheter is often considered at the beginning of a prolonged treatment programme, and insertion of a cvc will have short- and long-term implications for both the patient and his family. This stage in a patient's treatment can be stressful and the slightest concern can induce anxiety. It is therefore essential that the patient is well prepared and supported prior to, during the procedure, and following the catheter insertion.

Insertion of a catheter can affect the patient physically, psychologically, psychosexually and socially. As with any situation, each person will respond differently, and it is for this reason that preparation needs to be a well-planned process that is able to meet individual needs.

There are four main aims of patient preparation for a cvc. These are:

1. to gain informed consent for the catheter insertion
2. to reduce the risk of potential peri- and post-insertion complications

3. to promote maximum patient comfort
4. to ensure the patient understands the situation and is able to adjust to it.

To achieve a high quality of patient preparation, the nurse preparing the patient should have, at very least, a basic knowledge of the procedure and the implications for the patient and his family. This can be achieved by observing the procedure and also by discussing catheter insertion with other patients who have had a catheter placement previously. It may also be of benefit for the nurse to have a basic knowledge of how to use and care for the device, as this is information the patient will need to know.

Information must be available before patient preparation begins and should explain the type of device the patient is to have inserted, its estimated duration, and who is inserting it. For example, the patient will need to know whether the person inserting the device is a nurse specialist or a doctor, and where the procedure will take place, i.e. on the ward or in theatre. This will give the patient accurate, individualised information from an early stage.

Good patient preparation prior to the catheter insertion can take time. Catheter insertion for PN is usually a planned event and therefore arrangements can be made for preparation in advance. Although procedures vary in different hospitals, it is often the ward nurse who prepares the patient for the catheter insertion, as she is in the situation where she is able to assess the patient's individual preparatory needs.

Informed consent

Before the catheter can be inserted, the patient's consent is required. Consent is both a legal requirement and a tool for risk management (Buchanan 1995). It could be suggested that there are two types of consent:

1. consent, where the patient signs a document saying he agrees to the treatment; and
2. informed consent, where the patient is actively involved in the decision, and has an understanding of the relevant facts and information, enabling him to make an informed decision.

Informed consent is a legal standard providing the patient with all the information he requires, giving him the opportunity to be actively involved in decisions about his body and lifestyle. Informed consent is the right of every patient, according to 'The Patient's Charter' (Department of Health 1991). It is also part of the registered nurse's role to ensure that the patient has all the information he or she needs (UKCC 1992) to make an informed decision.

Sharing information may encourage the patient to ask questions and express his own wishes. Decisions based on these wishes allow the patient to maintain some control over events, which may help him achieve a higher level of self-care after catheter insertion. Active participation may promote wellbeing, which, when the patient faces a long treatment period, could be of benefit to both him and his family.

Having suggested that informed consent is preferable, it is important to consider how this can be achieved. Information involving the procedure, the uses of the device, postprocedural expectations, potential complications of the procedure and lifestyle implications are all issues that require addressing. Effective communication skills are essential if the patient is to be fully informed.

Barriers to effective communication

There are a number of barriers to informed consent (Box 5.1). As nurses we should be aware of these in order that they can be overcome.

We must be very aware of the language or terminology used. A patient who is relatively new to the hospital setting will be unfamiliar with the medical jargon that is often used. In contrast to this, a patient who is very knowledgeable about his disease and prescribed treatment may be familiar with the medical and nursing terms. Individuals whose first language is not English should also be considered and sources of support and information found for them, rather than allowing the language barrier to become a problem. Some hospitals may have a list of potential resources that may be of use in this situation.

It is also worth mentioning that some nurses may feel threatened by patients who have considerable knowledge regarding their disease and treatment. This, too, can be a barrier to informed consent, with the result that the patient may not receive the information he requires. Instead the patient may be avoided by the nurse, or it may be assumed that he possesses the relevant information.

It is important to remember that, as nurses, we are part of a multidisciplinary team, and although we may not always be able to answer the patient's questions, there will be other members of the team who can.

Attitudes of nurses can play a large role in the provision of information, as they may influence a patient's response. An example of this can be seen when a nurse is not convinced that the prescribed treatment is effective and conveys this message, sometimes unknowingly, to the patient.

Other barriers to informed consent include the sources of information,

Box 5.1   Barriers to effective communication
Language Jargon Attitude Lack of knowledge

particularly if only one source is used to prepare the patient as opposed to a variety of sources. A nurse less experienced in dealing with cvcs will not always be able to provide a clear picture of events; in this case an experienced member of the nursing team would be a more appropriate resource in the provision of this information.

What form the given information takes, and where information is given, could also present barriers, as many patients are unable to remember at this stage all that is said to them, and may not always have access to a nurse should they require additional information than that specified in a ward booklet. Suitable contents for a ward booklet are discussed later in this chapter.

The timing of information/education giving can also be important, as there are times when the patient may not be receptive to new information, particularly when he is feeling fatigued, nauseated, or in pain. This may also affect the patient's ability to understand.

The actual written permission associated with informed consent is usually part of the medical role. However, the whole team should be responsible for ensuring that the patient has been provided with the necessary information prior to giving consent.

PROVISION OF INFORMATION

Information about the catheter insertion procedure is given for many reasons: to inform, to educate and to reduce anxiety. Grahn (1996) suggests that information-giving should be an interactive process.

Information can be given verbally or in writing. When preparing the patient for catheter insertion, it is often better to give both kinds. This is because there may be a considerable amount of information to impart with regard to the actual procedure, the uses of cvcs, and care of the catheter following insertion. Written information will provide a reference for the patient and his family, both before and after catheter insertion.

Other sources of information may include videos; these can often be obtained from the catheter manufacturer. Videos have their advantages, and can be successfully used in group sessions where there are several patients having catheters placed. This may be an appropriate provision of information for a group of patients who are to receive home PN (HPN). However, not all patients wish to know the details of the procedure of catheter insertion! The videos selected should therefore provide the necessary information without the more technical aspects of the procedure.

Patients who have a catheter in place can also be a useful source of information when preparing other patients, particularly when there are no photographs or samples of catheters available. However, this is a resource that is not always available, and the patients who require cvc placement may be too ill to help or not always agreeable or appropriate.

If a patient with an existing cvc is available and willing to share his experiences with a new patient, it is worth taking time to consider your choice of candidate. Considering the sex of the patient who already has a catheter is also useful. Most women with subclavian catheters that exit above their breast will not appreciate being asked to expose themselves to male patients!

Patients receiving long-term PN can be a great source of information and will have a greater understanding of the procedure and its implications on lifestyle.

A clean, unsterile catheter will also provide an educational resource and give the patient the opportunity to handle a catheter and familiarise himself with the size and texture of the device.

Photographs can also be helpful, demonstrating to the patient what a catheter will look like when it is in place.

Ward booklet

Written information in the form of booklets is an ideal way of providing essential information on how the catheter is inserted, by whom and why. The booklet may have photographs to show what the device will look like. It should also give an indication of realistic expectations with regard to potential complications such as pain, catheter misdirection, pneumothorax and sepsis, as well as indications of potential implications of the catheter on an individual's lifestyle. This is particularly relevant for patients with HPN. An information booklet may also provide information on self-care of the device, relevant for HPN patients. However, there should be re-assurance that learning to care for a catheter is not a 'Do it yourself' experience and there is support available if the patient experiences difficulties. Details of the support that is available should be incorporated into the booklet.

When designing a booklet there are certain elements to consider, such as content readability and legibility (Arthur 1995). It should contain information that the patient will require, and needs to know. Production of a such a booklet can be expensive and therefore it is worth considering utilising booklets from other local or national sources. Other wards or departments who use cvcs frequently may have their own booklets that could be adapted for PN; for example gastroenterology, haematology, or the dietetic department. Alternatively, there may be national support groups that produce a booklet containing the information you and the patient require, e.g. the British Association of Parenteral and Enteral Nutrition (BAPEN). However, nationally produced booklets often contain general information and are produced for a variety of different specialities. Some individuals may benefit from information that is more specific to their requirements.

Individual requirements for information

To achieve individualised care, the patient's requirements of information should be assessed before information is imparted (McDermott 1995). This is especially important when considering the needs of someone who has had a cvc inserted previously, as opposed to those of someone who has not. It is also important to recognise and respect that some patients do not want a great deal of information; for these patients providing too much information may increase their fears.

The assessment of the patient's information needs should incorporate the patient's ability to understand the information, his age, his level of independence and who is going to care for the catheter. These considerations may affect what, how, and to whom information is given.

Following assessment of the patient's information requirements, it is then necessary to plan the information that is to be provided, when, and by whom it is going to be given. This is not always easy.

The information given is often restricted to what is available. However, despite the fact that there are a number of people within the multidisciplinary team who will be able to provide varying viewpoints to the patient, it is important for there to be consistency in the provision of information to avoid confusion.

The medical team will be able to discuss the rationale for having a catheter inserted, and will be able to provide information on treatment and possibly the duration of PN. The dietitian will be able to discuss with the patient dietetic aspects regarding PN, which are discussed elsewhere in this book (Ch. 8). Although team members such as the social worker and occupational therapist will not be directly involved in informing and educating the patient, they may have roles with regard to assistance with home support, should this be required.

Other people who are able to provide relevant information regarding the catheter and the insertion include the operator, who may be a clinical nurse specialist or a member of the medical team. It may also be important for a member of the community nursing team to be involved, particularly if she is going to be the principal supervisor of care in the community.

The timing of information and education is also important. Information should be provided at the earliest opportunity, thus giving the patient a reasonable period of time to comprehend the proposed therapy. The patient may wish to discuss this with his family and begin the process of adjustment.

McDermott (1995) suggests that to facilitate an effective exchange of information the patient must have symptoms of nausea or pain under control. It is also important to choose a place on the ward that is conducive to learning. A noisy bay, where there are frequent interruptions, is not the ideal place, and a side room may be more suitable.

When information is communicated, the nurse should be aware of information overload on the patient's part that may confuse the patient. To assess the patient's comprehension of information, and to pick up on areas of confusion, it may be advisable to receive feedback from the patient. This is particularly important for patients who will receive HPN, as it is essential that they fully understand the most basic principles of asepsis for successful administration of PN.

The patient and his family may need information repeated a number of times, particularly during the early stages of therapy. Open communication is essential if the patient is to benefit from the information/education process and will enable an honest and open relationship between patient and nurse. This is important because nurses are likely to have a predominant role in the provision of information/education, since they are often the coordinators of care and the patient's advocate.

Documentation is a vital part in the provision of information and education. It can provide a checklist for what information has been discussed, by whom and the outcome of the session. It can also provide an assessment of ongoing needs. Accurate documentation is essential when care is provided by a multidisciplinary team and will promote continuity and provide a framework to build on. Such documentation could be incorporated into care plans or a checklist could be developed within an existing local protocol.

PATIENT CONCERNS

This section considers the potential issues that the patient may identify regarding cvc insertion. It will often be the nurse who will suggest prospective ways of dealing with them. However, it is essential to remember that this is very general and care will need to be individualised in order for it to be effective.

Fear of the procedure

The patient may be worried about the actual insertion procedure. The patient's feelings must be respected and there are many ways in which anxiety and fears can be reduced with tact and diplomacy by the multidisciplinary team. Some patients require more information, especially those who are concerned with pain during the procedure, or who have never previously received sedation or been to the operating theatre. The type of additional information required by these patients often depends on the individual and which aspect of the procedure is concerning him.

Avoiding delays can also help reduce anxiety, as people may become very agitated whilst awaiting the procedure of catheter insertion. Reducing the wait is always advisable, but it is not always possible. In this situation it may be appropriate to utilise relaxation techniques, which may aid in the distraction of the patient prior to catheter insertion.

Reassurance will always be required before catheter insertion. Some patients may need more reassurance and support than others, but all should be encouraged to voice their fears and concerns. Reassurance from the nurse could be verbally, non-verbally, or merely by being a familiar person present during the procedure, as it is not always appropriate for a family member or friend to be present at this time. Insertion of a catheter may appear painful for the patient and may distress some people observing the procedure. The procedure may also involve some blood loss. There are a number of people who cannot tolerate this, which is another reason why it may not be appropriate for family to be present.

Anxiety

By providing information we are increasing the patient's knowledge, and for some this may induce anxiety. Although anxiety can be a normal reaction to change, and experience has suggested that a certain level of stress and anxiety may be required in order to retain information, it can have an adverse effect on some people's ability to retain information. For those patients suitable for HPN, profound anxieties regarding the responsibility of the cvc may present problems, in which case it may be advisable for an alternative carer to learn the skills involved in caring for the catheter.

Other possible reasons for anxiety prior to catheter insertion could understandably be fear of the procedure, as described above, especially if the patient feels that the catheter will 'sit in his heart'. The stress of the situation can be exacerbated, particularly if surgery is planned or chemotherapy is due to commence. Concern over the long-term implications on his lifestyle with the catheter in place, the treatment for which it will be inserted, together with fear of change in body image, are all possible causes of distress.

Anxiety can manifest itself in many ways including headaches, restlessness and an inability to sleep. It is important to observe the individual for such signs and support the patient during these episodes. Addressing psychological issues with the patient may have a positive effect on the patient's ability to cope after the procedure and may also help reduce future anxiety.

Assessment of the patient's level of anxiety requires a multidisciplinary approach. This will enable early and effective intervention with possible sedative measures during the insertion of the cvc. Effective assessment of anxiety can be aided through the use of open communication. This may include using both verbal and non-verbal communication, and relies upon the development of a trusting relationship between a group of nurses, the patient and his family. The opportunity to spend time with the patient without interruptions may also help. Open communication will also allow the nurse to assess the individual's coping mechanisms and help identify areas of support outside the hospital, such as family and friends.

Needle phobia

There seems to be little literature on the management of needle phobias within the acute hospital setting, but there are patients with a genuine fear of needles who require a cvc. The patient may express fear at the thought of needles and therefore nurses should observe the patient for non-verbal signs of fear or anxiety.

Identifying the fear of needles can take time, and involves detailed assessment. Patients will require support and understanding and should be encouraged to participate actively in decisions about how the problem is to be managed. The multidisciplinary team caring for the patient will be involved in creating options on how to manage the situation.

Detailed preparation prior to the catheter insertion for these patients will be required by the nursing and medical team. The use of a local anaesthetic cream prior to the procedure in order that a peripheral cannula can be placed painlessly will be appreciated by all patients. It may be appropriate for the needle phobic patient to have a cvc in theatre under anaesthetic, as opposed to a ward setting, respecting the patient's fears.

It is important to consider what type of catheter is to be used for a patient who experiences needle phobia. A device with an injectable port under the skin would not always be appropriate as it involves needles puncturing the skin each time therapy is commenced.

If the procedure is to take place on the ward, the patient will require intravenous sedation. Benzodiazepines have the effect of relaxing the patient and also have an amnesic effect, which can be very effective for this purpose. The dose of the drug required will depend on a variety of factors, e.g. the size of the patient, his past medical history, current clinical condition and other medications he may require. Drugs to be used for the procedure should be prescribed beforehand in order that delays can be avoided.

Intravenous sedatives require careful and accurate administration and therefore it is often useful to dilute such agents to a manageable and convenient solution. Diluting these agents will also eliminate the stinging sensation some patients experience when concentrated doses of drugs are administered via the venous route. When using benzodiazepines it is imperative that the reversal agent is available at all times, as one of the potential side-effects is that of respiratory depression. Should this occur, the reversal agent should be administered and emergency action taken by the medical and nursing team.

Physical aspects

There are a number of physical aspects involved in the preparation for insertion of the catheter, as the catheter may interfere with everyday activities that are taken for granted, such as wearing a car seat belt and wearing certain clothes comfortably. For these reasons it is important to include the patient in discussions of where and in which position the catheter will be most suitable. Such discussion encourages patient control over the situation and involves him in the decision-making process, and indicates that you see him as an individual. However, it is important to make the patient aware that it may not always be possible to place the catheter where he wants it, due to physical abnormalities, potential risks such as infection or stenosis of the vessel.

The medical team often have preferences for the choice of insertion site, but the patient's wishes should be respected and the rationale for the preferred site choice explained to him.

Choice of site

There are a number of considerations for the choice of site; this was discussed in greater depth in Chapter 4. The most important of these choices is probably the reason for the catheter insertion. The choice of site is usually the jugular, subclavian or femoral vein. Each site has its disadvantages and advantages, each carrying a potential risk of infection. Use of the subclavian site for catheter insertion is often preferred, as it has a lower infection risk in comparison to the jugular and the femoral approaches (Evans-Orr 1993). The femoral site can be particularly difficult to keep clean and, owing to the warm moist location, has a higher incidence of infection.

Parenteral nutrition carries its own risk of infection, so the aim is to reduce the overall risk. The risk of infection is especially important when the catheter is being inserted into the oncology/haematology patient receiving chemotherapy, as these patients may have a compromised immune system for prolonged periods.

The choice of insertion site also depends upon the condition of the vein into which the catheter is to be inserted. The vein condition may be affected if, for example, the patient has a tumour in that region of the body, a current infection, a thrombosis, or a pneumothorax (Elliot et al 1994). A previous catheter or surgery at the chosen site may also affect the integrity of the vein and surrounding tissue.

Other considerations that are relevant to individual patients when considering catheter placement for PN are their mobility and dexterity. This may affect their ability to care for the catheter, especially if it is in an awkward position, or if it will need frequent manipulation.

Considerations that the patient may mention include clothing irritation, especially with women's bra straps and position of a seat belt. It is necessary to identify these potential problems prior to catheter insertion, in order that the catheter is in a comfortable and manageable position for the patient. Methods of overcoming these problems would be for the catheter to be inserted into the left side of the chest wall, if the patient is a driver, or the the right-hand side if a non-driver or regular passenger. Identifying where bra straps lie before catheter insertion may also help. Communication of these details to the doctor or nurse specialist inserting the device is essential.

The scars that the catheter may leave behind may be of concern to the patient, before the catheter is inserted. Discussing and preparing the patient is necessary in order that he is aware of what measures can be taken to counteract this. The operator will be the person who will be best able to take this concern into consideration during the procedure. The choice of site is also a relevant issue here, especially if the patient wears low-cut clothing and does not wish the scars to be seen.

Having a catheter in place can lead to invasion of privacy which can cause great distress and embarrassment for the patient. It is desirable to consider this prior to catheter insertion, especially if the patient is to have a femoral line. Frequent access to a patient's groin area can be particularly embarrassing. The patient may therefore want to identify clothing that will reduce the risk of exposure of this area, before the catheter is inserted. However, it is sometimes impossible to overcome some problems with privacy in relation to femoral lines.

Self-care is a possible solution, but often in the early stages of PN the patient is too ill to achieve this. There is therefore likely to be a period where intrusion and embarrassment may be a problem.

Psychological aspects

The catheter does change the patient's appearance physically, both during its time in place and afterwards in the form of scars, however small. This may potentially affect the patient psychologically. It may also be a reminder of the underlying disease for which the catheter was inserted. All this can change the way a patient looks, feels and expresses himself, and how he considers others view him.

Changes in body image may affect an individual very deeply, which is why it is important to discuss the potential effects before the catheter is inserted. McDermott (1995) suggests that younger patients may find the change in body image harder to cope with than an older person; however, this is not always the case.

A catheter used for PN that exits from a breast, neck, or groin can affect the way the whole family communicates. The patient receiving HPN may feel that it inhibits his expression of sexuality with his partner, and it may

also be uncomfortable when cradling young children. This has consequences for the whole family. Body image is a very personal issue and
there are a number of people who feel uncomfortable discussing it. However, discussion can often bring concerns into the open and can assist
in finding methods of dealing with such problems. If a patient knows that
a nurse is willing to discuss sexuality before it becomes a problem, it may
be that if a problem occurs later, he may feel sufficiently relaxed to discuss
the issue without embarrassment.

Psychological issues can be difficult to address and the patient may need
counselling or further professional help. If the nurse does not feel best able
to cope with the issue of counselling, it is worth considering alternative
resources. These resources may include a nurse counsellor, nurse specialist
or a psychiatric nurse, but again, this will vary in each hospital.

Social aspects

Having a catheter in place can influence how a person dresses and functions during daily and social activities. It can also place great responsibility
on the patient, as he will need to care for it and maintain its function whilst
at home. The patient may be anxious about his loss of independence and
control over his life with a catheter in place. This may be even more of a
fear if this involves being connected to a machine for several hours a day,
possibly altering the activities of daily living. These issues should be
addressed prior to catheter insertion as the effects may, in some cases, be
minimised with planning.

Although it is not always easy to accommodate dress preferences when
deciding where to place a catheter, it is an element that could be incorporated into planning the catheter site, as previously mentioned.

It is essential to involve the patient in these issues and encourage him to
participate in all decisions so that he is able to maintain his independence
and control over the situation. The nurse is instrumental in encouraging
and educating the patient, or a family member to care for the device if the
patient is to be discharged whilst receiving PN. This will enable the patient
to achieve an optimum level of self-care and independence, within the constraints of having a catheter in place. However, taking the responsibility
for the catheter may be a source of anxiety (Clarke & Cox 1988). Therefore,
it is important that the patient is aware of what resources are available to
educate, help and support him if there is a problem, whilst in hospital or
at home. A reference booklet including useful telephone numbers can aid
this, as it is an easily accessible source of information to the patient.

Swimming is not always advisable when the HPN patient has a catheter
in place, although it may be possible to insert a catheter that is more
conducive to swimming if so wished. A catheter with an injectable port
located in a subcutaneous pocket, usually on the chest wall, as opposed to

one which has the tubing above the skin surface, may be more appropriate. However, it is worth remembering that there may be other reasons why activities such as swimming are not advisable, such as immunosuppression.

Holidays may also be important to the HPN patient, and this is an issue that may be mentioned prior to the catheter insertion. It may be that the patient will need additional equipment to take on holiday with him, particularly if foreign travel is considered. The patient may also need a doctor's letter.

There are ways of getting around the majority of concerns that the patient has, but we should be realistic about what can be offered to patients and why. As nurses we should be aware of the individual patient's concerns regarding his social activities in order that we are in a position to assess his needs and plan interventions that may help deal with them. It is important to be understanding of patient concerns as it is the patient who needs to live with the catheter, and not the multidisciplinary team!

As nurses we should be facilitative in order to meet the patient's needs and requirements, and be able and willing to provide continuing support and guidance.

PRACTICAL REQUIREMENTS

Site preparation

Preparation of the site of the catheter insertion can vary between hospitals. The removal of hair in the area is a very controversial issue and is often very much a personal preference of the operator. Hair removal normally includes the site of catheter insertion.

Removing hair has the advantages of allowing a better view of the area, which may assist the catheter insertion by limiting the risk of stray hairs obstructing access. It can also improve dressing adherence after the procedure, which promotes safe wound healing.

However, if the hair is to be removed then it is better to use clippers as opposed to a razor if possible, in an attempt to reduce the risk of infection from microabrasions. Clippers are recommended by the RCN Leukaemia and Bone Marrow Transplant Nursing Forum (1995). Other methods of removing hair include the use of depilatory cream. However, this can be time-consuming as a skin sensitivity test should be conducted prior to the procedure because there is a risk of an allergic reaction. A reaction to depilatory cream may compromise the patient and make the chosen site less accessible. This method of hair removal could also be expensive.

Peripheral venous access

Other aspects of patient care and preparation include ensuring that the patient has patent, peripheral venous access at an easily assessible site. This ensures that the sedation/anaesthetic and any blood products required prior to the procedure can be given easily and thus minimise distress to the patient.

Preoperative antibiotics

The use of preoperative antibiotics has also been a much-debated issue in the past, as some believe that using antibiotics will reduce the infection risk as a result of the procedure (Ranson et al 1990). This is a medical decision and, again, often depends upon the preference of the multidisciplinary team involved in the patient's care. Practice will vary in different hospitals' policies.

Medications

The patient's medications should also be taken into consideration before catheter insertion. For example, if the patient is on anticoagulants, measures to reduce the risk of bleeding may need to be considered. It may be that, in some rare situations, the HPN patient previously requiring anticoagulant therapy for other reasons will need possible anticoagulant dosage adjustment so that the risk of haemorrhage can be minimised.

In some areas, patients are commenced on low-dose warfarin, prior to catheter insertion. This continues for the lifespan of the catheter and is an attempt to reduce the risk of thrombosis (Bern et al 1990).

Blood analysis

Ideally, blood analysis should be performed 24 h before the procedure so that any abnormality detected in the results can be corrected. Normal parameters of coagulopathy are essential and therefore analysis should be arranged in good time prior to the proposed procedure.

The blood results that are most essential include a full blood count and clotting screen, although having the results of a urea and electrolyte sample may be of use in some situations. Having these results can reduce the risk of peri and post procedure complications such as bleeding, and measures can be taken to correct abnormal values before problems arise.

Although catheter insertion is sometimes referred to as minor procedure, in reality it can involve a severe degree of trauma and can be a life-threatening procedure in the hands of an inexperienced operator. Therefore, it is essential patient preparation ensures maximum patient stability prior to this procedure. Some patients will require blood products immediately prior to the procedure, especially if they are having coagulation problems or have a low platelet count. Time should be allowed for these blood products to be administered safely so that they can be effective in the control of bleeding.

Although the need for treatment is often decided by the medical team, the nurse has a role in bringing the current condition of the patient and recent blood results to the attention of the medical team. Therefore, the nurse should be aware of the rationale of necessary actions if not for herself, but for her patients, as many will question why they need additional treatment before the catheter is inserted and why it cannot wait until afterwards.

The full blood count will indicate the need for the patient to receive a blood transfusion, or more commonly platelets, particularly those patients with haematological disorders. These results will also give an indication of the septic state of the patient, and allow the operator to be fully aware of the patient's susceptibility to infection. The patient may also require fresh frozen plasma, or vitamin K, should coagulopathy demonstrate an abnormal result.

It is essential that the patient has any appropriate treatment necessary to ensure stability for cvc insertion in good time prior to the procedure. Interventions must not be rushed and must be carried out safely. Although better avoided, it is preferable to delay the procedure by a few minutes in order to give treatment safely.

HELPFUL HINTS IN PRE-CATHETER INSERTION

In order that the procedure runs smoothly, there are a number of pre-catheter checks that assist everyone involved, whether the procedure is to take place on the ward or in theatre.

- Ensure that the bed is functional, and that every function is in working order. The bed should have the ability to adopt the Trendelenburg position (Fig. 5.1). This position is preferred during catheter insertion as it allows the large vessels of the chest and neck to become engorged with blood. This aids cannulation and reduces the risk of an air embolism. The patient should be prepared that this position is necessary and reassured that it will be for a short time. Ideally the mattress should not be full of air, as this can be an unstable surface for the procedure. It also may not deflate rapidly in the event of an emergency.
- Adequate lighting in the area is essential and the bedside light should be checked to ensure it is in working order.
- A pulse oximeter should be available throughout the procedure. This will provide reassurance to the operator and will aid in an immediate assessment of oxygen levels and cardiac rate.
- Ensure that the patient consent is signed before the patient is sedated!
- Allow time for the blood results to return to the ward and ensure that

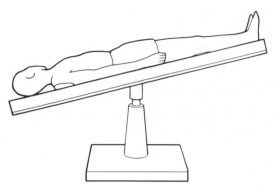

Figure 5.1   Trendelenburg position. Reproduced from Rosen M, Latto P, Ng S 1992 Handbook of percutaneous central venous catheterisation 2E. WB Saunders, London, with permission.

the operator has seen these before the procedure commences. If the patient is going to theatre, the anaesthetist may have visited the patient, but may not have seen the blood results – ensure they are easily accessible. A good place to put them is on a piece of paper, clearly labelled, on the front of the medical notes.

• The operator will need an assistant, if the procedure is to be performed on the ward, so ensure that there is someone available.

• Ensure that the drugs to be used during the procedure are prescribed and available, with any necessary reversal agents or emergency drugs readily available also.

• Emergency equipment and a chest drainage set should also be readily accessible.

Catheter insertion is often a good time for observation and learning for both nursing and junior medical staff. If anyone wishes to observe, the patient's consent should be gained. The operator should also be asked for verbal consent beforehand. Considering details in advance may prevent delays and reduce the risk of confusion in the event of an emergency.

CONCLUSION

The result of good nursing care prior to the catheter insertion should be a well-prepared, calm, consenting patient who is aware of the potential complications and implications on his lifestyle. The patient should also be informed as to why the catheter is being inserted, what support is available to him during its placement, and the potential complications associated with central venous access. The patient would hopefully have begun the process of adjustment to the current situation.

Case Study 5.1 illustrates how careful and thorough preparation, with

Case Study 5.1

Alice, a young woman with short gut due to Crohn's disease, and receiving PN, was admitted to the department of gastroenterology for a catheter change owing to catheter damage. Previous catheter insertions had been traumatic, with little information provided and devices inappropriately sited. In view of her experiences and her dislike of the damaged catheter and its performance, it was decided to insert a new type of device.

Despite a great deal of new information to take on board at this stage, preparation for the catheter insertion began the day she arrived on the ward, in a quiet side room. Alice was given an explanation of what the new device was, how it worked, and why it was appropriate for her treatment. She was able to hold a clean catheter, to familiarise herself with the feel of it, and discuss the procedure and the device with another patient. She was also given an information booklet to read and encouraged to ask questions when she thought of them. Her questions were answered by the multidisciplinary team caring for her, which also included the nurse specialist who would insert the catheter.

Detailed discussion regarding Alice's lifestyle, the types of clothes she preferred were considered by the specialist nurse and the patient. It was decided during this short visit that the device would be inserted in the subclavian region and on Alice's right-hand side, as she did not drive. The chosen area also meant that the catheter would be supported by her bra and not be in the line of her bra strap. Alice was happy about this position as she also felt it would not be easily visible to others. Alice said that she understood why she needed the device and was relieved that she would not require needles in her arm once the device was in position. However, she did express fear of the procedure itself and caring for the device, as it sounded complicated and differed from the device she had been used to.

Both the nursing and medical staff were able to talk through the procedure with Alice and her family, and reassure her that she would be sedated and remember nothing of the procedure. Another patient was also able to offer support and reassurance that she would feel very little, apart perhaps from the installation of the local anaesthetic which would sting momentarily. She was also happier knowing that a familiar ward nurse would be present during the procedure.

The procedures involved in caring for the catheter were explained to Alice, but she was reassured that she would not be expected to do this until she felt ready, and that she would be taught in greater detail when the catheter was in place and the effects of the sedative agent dispersed. It was reiterated that she would be able to carry out the catheter care with assistance when she began learning, and that when she went home there would always be someone on the ward to offer advice over the telephone. Alice signed the consent the day before the procedure, having been fully informed about potential complications by the operator. Her coagulopathy and haematology were checked at this time.

The results suggested that the low-dose anticoagulation Alice had received whilst receiving HPN, to reduce the risk of thrombin formation at the tip of the catheter, had resulted in her blood clotting being slightly prolonged. It was decided to administer some fresh frozen plasma to aid her clotting during the procedure.

Alice had her catheter inserted without peri- or postoperative complications as planned.

concern for the patient's wishes, can make the procedure of cvc insertion more agreeable for the patient and complication-free.

This chapter has considered a number of issues associated with pre-catheter insertion, and it may seem that there are many potential problems involved. It is important to point out that a large proportion of individuals who have a cvc inserted do not experience any of these problems, but the potential for them to occur is·always there. The nurse has a vital role in minimising these by facilitating the majority of the issues discussed in this chapter.

REFERENCES

Arthur VAM 1995 Written patient information: a review of the literature. Journal of Advanced Nursing 21:1081–1086
Bern MM, Lokick JJ, Wallach SR et al 1990 Very low doses of warfarin can prevent thrombosis in central venous catheters. Annals of Internal Medicine 112:423–428
Buchanan M 1995 Enabling patients to make informed decisions. Nursing Times 91(18):27–29
Clarke J, Cox E 1988 Heparinisation of Hickman catheters. Nursing Times 84 (15):52–53
Department of Health 1991 The patient's charter. HMSO, London
Elliot TSJ, Faroqui MH, Armstrong RF, Hanson GC 1994 Guidelines for good practice in central venous catheterisation. Journal of Hospital Infection 28:163–176
Evans-Orr M 1993 Issues in the management of percutaneous central venous catheters. Nursing Clinics of North America 28(4):913–919
Grahn G 1996 Patient information as a necessary therapeutic intervention. European Journal of Cancer Care 5(suppl 1):7–8
McDermott MK 1995 Patient education and compliance issues associated with access devices. Seminars in Oncology Nursing 11(3):221–226
Ranson MR, Oppenhiem BA, Jackson A, Kamthan AG, Scarff H 1990 Double blind placebo controlled study of vancomycin prophylaxis for central venous catheter insertion in cancer patients. Journal of Hospital Infection 15:95–102
Royal College of Nursing Leukaemia and Bone Marrow Transplant Nursing Forum (1995) Skin tunnelled catheters. Guidelines for care, 2nd edn. RCN, Harrow
UKCC 1992 Code of Professional Conduct for nurse, midwife, and health visitor, 2nd edn. United Kingdom Central Council, London

FURTHER READING

Barraclough J 1994 Cancer and emotion 2nd edn. J Wiley, Chichester
Daniels LE 1995 The physical and psychosocial implications of central venous devices in cancer patients – a review of the literature. Journal of Cancer Care 4:141–145
Dennis KE 1990 Patients' control and the information imperative: clarification and confirmation. Nursing Research 39(3):162–166
Nichols KA 1993 Psychological care in physical illness, 2nd edn. Chapman & Hall, London
North G, Margree G, Roe M 1996 Guidelines for producing patient information literature. Nursing Standard 10(47):46–48
Price B 1990 Body image: nursing concepts and care. Prentice Hall, London.
Radcliffe S 1993 Preoperative information: the role of the ward nurse. British Journal of Nursing 2(6):305–309

6

The insertion of a central venous catheter for parenteral nutrition

Helen Hamilton

Introduction
Indications for central venous
  cannulation
Patient assessment and information
Patient preparation for central venous
  cannulation
Techniques and equipment

Factors influencing the choice of
  method of central venous cannulation
Percutaneous and peripheral catheter
  placement
Avoiding complications in the use of
  cvcs used for PN
Discussion

INTRODUCTION

The aim of this chapter is to help nursing and medical teams consider how best to insert a central venous catheter (cvc) safely and effectively for the reliable administration of parenteral nutrition (PN). Central venous cannulation has in the past been associated with increased infection and other complications. However, an experienced and well-informed nursing and medical team can ensure that such complications are minimised by using a structured and systematic approach (Traeger et al 1986). The potential for complications associated with cvc insertion is reduced if the patient requiring PN is adequately assessed and prepared both physically and psychologically.

INDICATIONS FOR CENTRAL VENOUS CANNULATION

Central venous cannulation is carried out for four main reasons; these are listed in Box 6.1. This book concentrates on the administration of PN.

As discussed in Chapter 4, the rationale and predicted duration of PN will often determine which cvc should be used. An awareness of the patient's clinical condition provided by the nursing and medical team will aid the operator in selecting the safest and most appropriate cvc for each patient.

Box 6.1   Indications for central venous cannulation

- Emergency venous access
- Measurement of central venous pressure
- Delivery of medications recommended for central venous administration, i.e. inotropic agents, chemotherapy and high-dose antibiotic therapies
- Administration of PN

PATIENT ASSESSMENT AND INFORMATION

Screening and assessment of the patient's current clinical and nutritional status aids in the identification of patients who will benefit from the administration of artificial nutrition via the central venous route, and may therefore reduce morbidity. The many components of assessment are listed in Box 6.2. Venous access is only considered after an assessment has been made for the purpose of PN and its anticipated duration.

The patient may have many anxieties associated with the insertion of a cvc. Discussion with the patient and an assessment of his tolerance to pain, plus any other concerns he may have regarding the procedure, provides the operator with the opportunity to allay apprehensions the patient may be harbouring. For example, prior knowledge of needle phobia, deep anxiety regarding sedation or the fear of lying flat will provide a helpful assessment for the operator and the patient. Discussion of these concerns engenders a feeling of trust between the patient and the operator, which will help to make the insertion of a cvc as relaxed as possible (see Ch. 5).

Clinical assessment

The assessment of clinical status in each patient is important, and will ensure that stability is maximised prior to the insertion of a cvc. It is essential that the operator acquires a detailed history when considering the insertion of a cvc, as this knowledge will help reduce the potential for complications often associated with the device. Information regarding previous medical problems such as surgery, asthma, congestive cardiac failure, and fractures involving the clavicle may affect the operator's decision as to which approach is made to central venous cannulation.

An assessment protocol may assist in ensuring the stability of the patient prior to the attainment of central venous access for administration of medication via the vascular system (Hamilton & Fermo 1998).

Box 6.2 Recommendations for assessment of patients requiring central venous catheterisation for parenteral nutrition

---

- Establish the indication for central venous cannulation
- Conduct an accurate clinical examination
- Conduct a detailed laboratory assessment
- Conduct a complete cardiovascular assessment
- Conduct a detailed neurological assessment
- Conduct a complete allergy assessment
- Conduct a complete nutritional assessment
- Obtain detailed patient information
- Obtain peripheral vascular access

Laboratory assessment

Haematological stability, i.e. agreed parameters of the clotting profile, platelet count, etc., will ensure haematological stability during venous cannulation. Local protocol will determine the accepted parameters of coagulopathy. A suggested range for the purpose of cvc insertion would be activated partial thromboplastin time (APTT) 22–38 s, prothrombin time (PT) 12–16 s. These values are an important indication of the patient's ability to form fibrin, which reduces the risk of bleeding. This safety measure is vital and there may be serious repercussions if precautions are not taken to gain patient stability prior to the insertion of a cvc.

It is the responsibility of the medical team and the operator to ensure that safe limits are met prior to commencing this invasive vascular procedure. Many patients, for example those with haematological malignancy, may require blood products to ensure optimum stability prior to central venous cannulation. Adequate quantities of blood products should always be planned and made available should the need arise. A local protocol for reduction or cessation of anticoagulant therapy prior to cannulation of major vessels may also reduce the risk of adverse haematological complications.

PN should never be considered as emergency treatment and therefore every effort should be made by the referring medical team to stabilise the patient's haematological and biochemical status prior to the insertion of a cvc.

Septic profile

An elevated white blood cell count or elevated temperature will raise the question of whether a permanent tunnelled cvc is appropriate in the septic patient. Advice from the microbiology team will help in deciding which type of venous device and which site of placement will be the most appropriate for the septic patient.

Current inflammatory markers should also be noted, and where elevated the question of central venous access should be addressed. Peripheral venous access may provide an alternative until patient stability is achieved, thus reducing the risk of compromising the septic patient further.

Cardiovascular assessment

Cardiovascular stability is certainly desirable, but it is not always possible when the insertion of a cvc is proposed. Careful assessment of the patient will establish the underlying cause of arrhythmias and, in some cases, simple correction of biochemical abnormalities will resolve the problem. However, a more complex cardiac arrhythmia will require advice from the cardiologist prior to the insertion of the cvc. An alternative to central venous access, using a peripheral approach, may be necessary until the patient's stability is ensured.

In addition, basic functions should be sufficiently stable. Sinus cardiac rhythm, normotensive and general haemodynamic stability will minimise complications occurring in the already compromised patient.

It is important to note that hypovolaemia, sepsis or shock are contra-indications for the insertion of a cvc, owing to the already compromised condition of the patient. However, in an emergency situation, to aid the operator in the insertion of a cvc in a hypovolaemic patient, the medical team may feel it necessary to administer additional fluid or colloid to aid in the adequate filling of the intravascular system. However, extreme care must be taken in the administration of additional fluid to the fluid-sensitive patient. Expert advice must be sought when faced with this situation in the cardiac patient, avoiding fluid overload that would possibly compromise the patient's clinical condition. A negative fluid balance and low central venous pressure may be preferable for the wellbeing of some patients. However, this may create operational difficulties associated with the location and cannulation of the appropriate vessel.

Patients with cardiac conditions will require specific assessment by the cardiology team. The potential for complications associated with central venous cannulation will be reduced when a team approach is adopted in the preparation of the patient prior to the insertion of a cvc. In some cardiac conditions, where the patient's cardiac stability is in doubt, a surgical or radiological approach to central venous cannulation may be preferable to percutaneous insertion. The method of insertion and type of central venous access will be determined according to individual patient requirements. This situation will require experienced judgment by the operator and the team responsible for the patient.

Respiratory assessment

The majority of patients requiring central venous access may be described as seriously ill, and are often not only cardiovascularly unstable, but may also experience respiratory difficulty and/or failure. This may be due to sepsis, sputum retention and/or electrolyte or fluid imbalance. To an operator experienced in the assessment of the patient requiring venous access, these factors would provide valuable information regarding the safest and most appropriate venous access required in the compromised patient.

Assessment of the patient's respiratory function will determine the patient's current respiratory status and provide the operator with information that may prevent a deterioration in the overall condition of the patient requiring central venous access. Abnormal respiratory function may influence the operator's choice of site for venous access and the technique of insertion for the cvc. Patients with asthma, emphysema or pleural effusion may be unable to tolerate lying flat or adopting the head-down (Trendelenburg) position (see Fig. 5.1) during the insertion of a cvc. A peripheral approach, either in the use of a peripherally inserted central catheter (PICC), or simply peripheral venous access, may be a more suitable method for this group of patients. Central venous access may be considered when the patient has a stable respiratory status.

Respiratory status is particularly important when considering the ventilated patient, who is at a greater risk of pneumothorax during the insertion of a cvc, owing to hyperinflation of the lungs. An experienced operator is particularly important in this group of patients, where accidental pneumothorax may severely jeopardise the patient's condition.

Vascular assessment

A structured and systematic approach to the examination of the patient prior to gaining venous access will aid in establishing the patency of the patient's venous system, thus reducing the risk of venous stenosis and unnecessary scarring of the patient's body.

Thrombosis, stenosis and anatomical anomalies may present difficulties for the operator when venous selection is being considered. Careful and detailed visual clinical examination of the thorax and upper limbs may reveal the presence of a dilated collateral venous circulation of the chest wall, limbs and neck. This may demonstrate the presence of thrombosis or possible stenosis as a result of previous therapies via the central venous route.

Interventional radiology or sophisticated vascular ultrasound may provide a useful diagnostic aid in the vascular assessment of the patient. This may reduce the risk of potential thrombotic complications or damage to the venous and arterial systems.

The venous network of any patient, and in particular the renal patient, is very precious and may often be required intermittently for life. The need for preserving and respecting these vessels should be paramount in the assessment process prior to gaining venous access in any patient.

Despite the vast numbers of veins in the body, only a few are considered suitable for central venous access, as discussed in Chapter 4 (see Fig. 4.1). A diagram of the venous circulation of each patient, with documentation following each insertion, can aid a new operator in the decision of which vessel to cannulate. This is particularly helpful when there is no dedicated central line insertion service.

Neurological assessment

Neurological considerations are important in the patient suffering from head injury or any other pertinent neurological condition. The Trendelenburg position (see Fig. 5.1), adopted by the patient for the insertion of cvc, may present a problem, with the likelihood of increasing intracranial pressure. In this instance, an alternative approach to venous access may be necessary.

A PICC or peripherally administered PN will avoid the potential hazard of raised intracranial pressure in this group of patients if suitable venous vessels are available.

Allergy assessment

During the clinical examination of the patient the question of allergy should be addressed. This is particularly important as skin cleansing agents, sedatives or certain dressings may not only cause unnecessary discomfort to the allergic patient, but may also possibly present a problem if an allergy to sedation or local anaesthetic is a factor.

Patients may not appreciate the association of previous allergies and the proposed procedure. A process of elimination performed either by the nursing team or the operator will limit risks involving allergies associated with cvc insertion.

Drug sensitivity is pertinent, particularly when the cvc is to be inserted percutaneously and a sedative agent is to be administered. Tolerance to sedation generally may be an unknown quantity, particularly in the elderly patient.

Nutritional assessment

Detailed nutritional assessment should be performed by the Nutrition Support Team (NST), in particular the dietitian who will be responsible for the assessment of the patient's nutritional requirements while considering the patient's current clinical condition. Detailed discussion regarding nutritional assessment will be found in Chapter 8.

Following nutritional assessment it may be that PN may only be required for a short period of time, i.e. 5–10 days. In this case a peripheral venous cannula or PICC may be more appropriate. Nutritional assessment and the method by which it is administered may well influence the choice of which type of catheter is to be inserted.

PREPARATION FOR CENTRAL VENOUS CANNULATION
Patient preparation

Once a decision has been made to proceed with central venous cannulation, the patient must be correctly prepared. There are many aspects to this preparation, as outlined in Box 6.3.

The patient will have been examined during the initial assessment, as described above, and patient stability and coagulopathy determined.

Box 6.3   Patient preparation for tunnelled central venous cannulation

---

- Patient examination
- Patient stability
- Patient information/education
- Patient consent
- Stable coagulopathy
- Peripheral venous access
- Body image issues

Gaining central venous access is a high-risk procedure and patient safety must be of paramount importance. Therefore, in order to avoid unnecessary complications, a detailed assessment of the clinical state of the patient must be carried out before central venous cannulation is attempted. Patient information and education, consent, coagulopathy and body image issues have been discussed in detail in Chapter 5.

Whether tunnelled central venous access is to be gained surgically or by a percutaneous approach, in many cases the patient will require peripheral venous access prior to this procedure. As noted in Chapter 5, temporary venous access should be readily patent for the administration of intravenous sedation or emergency drugs, if required. Peripheral venous access should be clearly visible with no evidence of thrombophlebitis or infection around the cannulation site. Many sedatives can be irritating to the vein, causing discomfort during administration. Once the planned central venous access is gained, the effect of sedation diminished, and the position of the cvc checked and deemed satisfactory, the peripheral cannula may be removed.

Preparation of operating venue and equipment

Any cvc insertional approach requires a clean area where a high standard of asepsis is practised, thus limiting infection. Minimisation of infection will also largely depend on two issues: the experience of the operator, and the absence of bacteria on the patient's skin.

As with many practical clinical procedures, success can be evaluated by the performance and reliability of the equipment used and the experience of the operator. Frustrations can be minimised by thoroughly checking all the equipment to be used and ensuring that emergency equipment is readily available prior to the commencement of the procedure. If the percutaneous method of insertion is chosen, then this procedure may either be performed at the patient's bedside or in a dedicated clean area.

Lighting

Adequate natural light will be beneficial to the operator. In the event that natural light is insufficient, a reliable portable light source must be found.

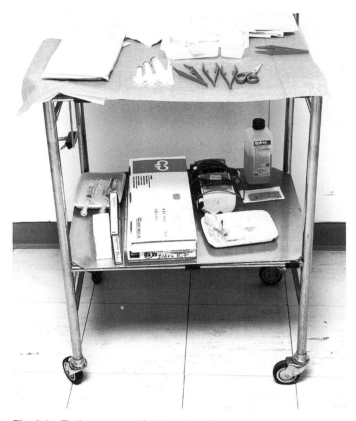

Fig. 6.1   Trolley prepared for insertion of a cvc.

The operator responsible for the insertion of the cvc should also be responsible for the aseptic preparation of the operating trolley (Fig. 6.1). Thorough checking of all equipment such as oxygen, suction and oximeter (a small device for measuring oxygen saturation applied to the finger or toe) will facilitate regular assessment of the patient's peripheral oxygenation. Any drugs that may be required, e.g. benzodiazepines or local anaesthetic, also become the responsibility of the appointed operator and assistant.

Space

It is important to ensure that adequate space is available for the operator and assistant during the insertion of a cvc. The operator, assistant and nurse will normally be the team involved in the insertion of a cvc. However, more often than not, particularly in teaching hospitals, students may also wish to observe the procedure. As mentioned in Chapter 5, these considerations should be planned in advance.

TECHNIQUES AND EQUIPMENT

With the variety of suitable products available for the delivery of PN, selection is often made easier once the operator is defined, particularly if the role is dedicated to the insertion of cvc for the purpose of PN. The operator will become adept and confident in the chosen technique, thus reducing the risk of serious complications associated with central venous cannulation.

However, an experienced operator may not always be available, and the product may be selected for the less experienced operator, encouraging a safer technique (Editorial 1986). In either case the choice of equipment and the method to be used should be considered with care. Options include:

- catheter through the needle
- catheter over the needle
- catheter through a cannula
- catheter over a guidewire
- subcutaneous port.

Catheter through the needle (Fig. 6.2)

This technique was popular some years ago but is rarely used now. Although relatively simple to use, it has the advantage of the needle entering the vein without the catheter coming into contact with the skin and subcutaneous tissue. The catheter is encased within a sterile sheath, enabling a non-touch technique during the insertion process.

However, due to the design, in that the needle is larger than the catheter, oozing from the venotomy may cause swelling at the puncture site. Another disadvantage is the potential for the catheter to shear should it be pulled against the needle. Severe damage in this way may cause complete shearing of the catheter, resulting in the proximal end of the catheter advancing freely into the vascular system.

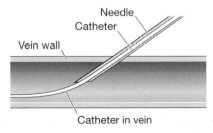

Fig. 6.2   Catheter through the needle.

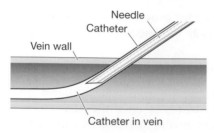

Fig. 6.3   Catheter over the needle.

Catheter over the needle (Fig. 6.3)

This device was designed in an attempt to overcome the problems associated with the previous method. In this design the needle is found within the catheter and presents no risk of the catheter shearing into the vascular circulation. In addition, the venotomy site is smaller, therefore reducing the risk of oozing around the cannulation site.

The main disadvantage to this device is the occasional damage caused by the rigid tip of the catheter as it enters the vein and the needle is withdrawn.

Catheter through a cannula (Fig. 6.4)

This technique was designed to utilise the advantages of the previous two methods while overcoming their disadvantages. Venepuncture is achieved with a syringe attached to a cannula with the needle inside. The cannula must be stiff and sufficiently sharp to pass through the skin and the wall of the vein. Once successful venepuncture is achieved the needle is removed, leaving the cannula within the vein and permitting advancement of the catheter into the vascular system.

Specific disadvantages remain. Due to the size of the cannula the catheter is smaller and may allow oozing from the larger venotomy site. In addition, the syringe must be disconnected from the catheter, thus creating a small

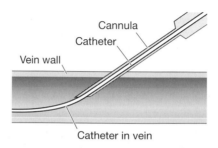

Fig. 6.4   Catheter through a cannula.

risk of air embolism. However, despite these potential complications, this method of cannulation has been used successfully for PN over varying durations.

Catheter over the guidewire, with or without a vein dilator and splittable sheath (Fig. 6.5)

This type of device is particularly suitable for the subclavian and jugular sites of insertion where the catheter is advanced over the Seldinger wire into the vein of choice. The Seldinger wire is flexible with a J-shaped tip to ensure that puncture of the vein is avoided.

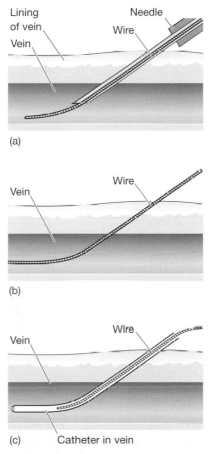

(a)

(b)

(c)   Catheter in vein

Fig. 6.5   Catheter over the guidewire (non-vein dilator technique). (a) Wire entering through the needle. (b) Wire lying in the vein. (c) Wire withdrawn after the catheter has been advanced over the wire, leaving the catheter in the vein.

Using this technique the vein is cannulated and a wire advanced through the needle. Once the wire is correctly positioned the needle is removed, leaving the wire in position within the venous system. The catheter is measured against the patient's chest, to ensure that the tip of the catheter will ultimately lie in the superior vena cava.

To avoid the risk of air entering the venous circulation, the catheter is lubricated/flushed with heparinised saline and threaded over the wire into the vein and advanced into the final position. The Seldinger wire is then removed and the catheter aspirated to ensure venous position.

This technique is used routinely for the insertion of multilumen and single-lumen catheters, reducing the risk of damage to deep structures and air embolism – a recognised complication with the use of through the cannula devices.

When the method includes a vein dilator and splittable sheath, these will be advanced over the Seldinger wire into the venous system. The wire and vein dilator will be removed, permitting the catheter to be advanced into the splittable sheath and into the venous circulation. The sheath is split, and the catheter slowly advanced until the entire catheter is inserted into the vein, whereupon the sheath splits away entirely.

To minimise the risk of infection when a cvc is inserted for the purpose of PN, it is widely considered that subcutaneous tunnelling will reduce catheter-related sepsis by delaying the tracking of skin-related organisms from the exit site of the tunnel to the venous circulation (Freedmans & Bosserman 1993). However, irrespective of advanced modern practice and materials, only strict aseptic technique and care associated with cvc management will ensure catheter-related sepsis is kept to a minimum (Elliott et al 1994).

Catheter over a guidewire

This method of cannulating the great vessels of the chest and neck is used extensively in the field of radiology, often using very fine wires to navigate the complex venous and arterial network. Whether used for a peripheral or central approach to central venous access, the guidewire method is usually a successful technique in the hands of an experienced operator.

However, guidewires are not without their hazards and have been known to puncture central venous walls and cardiac tissue, causing serious complications such as cardiac tamponade. For safety reasons a J-shaped type of Seldinger wire is advisable, in an attempt to avoid such complications. Guidewires have been known to knot within the vascular system as a result of the often tortuous course of venous structures.

Cvcs can also be inserted surgically or radiologically, under X-ray guidance. Patients may also express a wish to have the procedure performed under general anaesthesia. Whichever method is chosen, the same prin-

---

Box 6.4   Advantages and disadvantages of surgical placement of cvcs

Advantages
- Less experienced operator possible with some supervision
- Sterile area
- More conducive to needle-phobic patients
- Screening facilities available
- Patient stability ensured, prior to returning to ward

Disadvantages
- Theatre arrangement time-consuming
- Cost incurred from theatre time + anaesthetic and surgical costs
- Less opportunity for patient and operator to discuss position of cvc
- Increased potential for cancellation
- Increased patient anxiety

---

ciples of assessment and preparation apply. The advantages and disadvantages of surgical techniques of catheter insertion are listed in Box 6.4.

FACTORS INFLUENCING THE CHOICE OF METHOD OF CENTRAL VENOUS CANNULATION

A number of factors influence the choice of site for central venous cannulation. These are listed in Box 6.5.

Patient's clinical condition

As previously mentioned, the patient's clinical stability must be assured. PN should never be considered an emergency treatment and therefore careful preparation of the patient in every sense will guarantee the safe insertion of a cvc for PN. Biochemistry, clotting profile and other haematology should all be within acceptable parameters before cannulation is attempted.

In the event that the patient is clinically unstable, peripheral nutrition is always an option until such time that clinical stability of the patient is gained.

Box 6.5   Factors that influence the choice of method of central venous cannulation

- Patient's clinical condition
- Patency and availability of the great vessels of the neck and thorax
- Clotting profile
- Current venous access sites
- Catheter-related sepsis
- Available operator
- Operator's expertise
- Allergic factors
- Needle phobia

In many centres a surgical approach to gain central venous access in the provision of PN is routine. However, not all patients will be sufficiently stable to undergo a general anaesthetic. In this situation it may be more appropriate for peripheral access to be considered until clinical stability is reached and a permanent access device placed.

Patency and availability of the great vessels of the neck and thorax

The ultimate deciding factor when selecting a vascular device for the delivery of PN is the availability of a suitable vein. In many of the patients requiring this method of nutrition, previous hospital admissions involving PN, chemotherapy or antibiotic therapy may have resulted in what would have been ideal venous access becoming thrombosed or damaged, making future cannulation of the same vessel impossible. It is therefore extremely important to remember that an operator may be limited in the choice of venous access by the quality of the veins and the equipment available.

Due to venous anomaly, disease process or tumour affecting the venous anatomy of the chest, it may not be possible to obtain central venous access using a subclavian approach. An alternative approach may include a PICC, thus avoiding the affected area. Hence, alternatives may have to be considered, always with the patient's understanding and agreement.

Clotting profile

This has been discussed earlier in the section on laboratory assessment.

Current venous access sites

Venous access used for other purposes should be assessed by the operator. In some cases, for example where an internal jugular vein is used for clear fluids or antibiotics, this access may have to be removed if the subclavian vein is the only available site for PN, for fear of contamination. Ideally a vein to be used for PN should have no other agent administered via its route. This will maximise the life and performance of the device and reduce the risk of infection and damage to the selected vessel.

Catheter-related sepsis

This is common if a strict aseptic technique is not respected in the management of any intravenous therapy. Whatever the underlying cause of infection may be, it is wise not to insert a cvc until bacteriological stability of the patient is assured. The microbiologist can be of great assistance when advising on the timing of this procedure so as to avoid compromising the malnourished patient still further.

Expertise of the operator

As discussed in Chapter 4, the expertise of the operator is paramount in the insertion of any cvc. The success of any attempt at venous cannulation stems from the theoretical and practical experience of the operator (Box 6.6). However, despite most anaesthetists having considerable experience, with arm and neck veins in particular, no operator will be familiar with all techniques and the equipment available.

The inexperienced operator should select a technique that is essentially safe, although possibly yielding a lower success rate (Box 6.7). If a particular route is absolutely indicated, the assistance of an experienced operator should be sought. Temporary nutritional support can be provided to the malnourished patient until expert operating skills are available to insert sophisticated and often complex venous access.

Centres providing a nutritional support service will often have a dedicated team of operators inserting cvcs for this specific purpose with a standard insertion method. The method employed to gain venous access for PN will often be determined by the operator's success in either the peripheral or central approach and the complications associated with both. The experience of the operator is therefore an important factor in the success and safety of the cannulation of veins to be used for PN (Bo-Linn et al 1982, Sznajder et al 1986).

Whichever technique is to be used, it is essential that the patient has been adequately prepared and is in optimal condition prior to the insertion of a cvc that is to be used for PN. It should be remembered that commencement of PN is not an emergency and the insertion of a cvc for this purpose should always be planned and performed in a structured fashion with consideration for possible future venous access.

Box 6.6   Qualities necessary for the operator

- Ability to access the patient requiring central venous access for PN
- Practical expertise
- Theoretical knowledge
- Recognition and management of complications

Box 6.7   Factors to aid in selection of technique

- Patient stability
- Experience of available operator
- Operator's success for peripheral and central cannulation
- Suitability of technique in relation to patient's age, clinical state and lifestyle (particularly if catheter will be used for home PN)
- Complication risk

Box 6.8   Factors to consider when selecting equipment

- Familiar product
- Availability
- Suitability of catheter material for individual patients
- Cost
- Repair equipment availability

Equipment available

Equipment selection may be influenced by many factors (see Box 6.8). With the variety of suitable products available for the delivery of PN, selection is often made easier once the operator is defined, particularly if his role is dedicated to the insertion of cvcs for the purpose of PN. The operator will become adept and confident in the chosen catheter and method of cvc insertion, thus reducing the risk of serious complications associated with central venous cannulation.

The choice of catheter material, the method of insertion and subsequent management should be considered with care. However, one of the most important factors in the administration of PN is the use of a dedicated cvc, thus limiting the risk of infection and blockage which can occur if the catheter is used for multiple purposes. Other factors when considering the type of catheter to be used should also include the anticipated duration of PN, particularly when prolonged periods of artificial nutrition are anticipated.

The considerations that must be afforded to selection of the appropriate catheter are discussed in more detail in Chapter 4.

Allergic factors and needle phobia

Allergy assessment has been discussed earlier in the chapter. Needle phobia is discussed in detail in Chapter 5.

PERCUTANEOUS AND PERIPHERAL CATHETER PLACEMENT

This section describes in detail the percutaneous insertion of a cvc and the insertion of a PICC.

Tunnelled catheter placement using a percutaneous, infraclavicular approach

The advantages and disadvantages to using a percutaneous infraclavicular approach to cvc insertion are listed in Box 6.9. Before inserting the cvc

---

Box 6.9 Advantages and disadvantages of percutaneous infraclavicular placement of a cvc

Advantages
- Experienced operator reduces infection and other insertion-related complications
- Reduced cost due to avoidance of theatre time and anaesthetic
- Possible day case, alleviating bed occupancy
- Less stressful to the patient, unless needle phobic, when surgical placement is preferable
- Immediate cvc placement if patient's condition permits plus the availability of experienced operator
- Familiar nursing staff

Disadvantages
- Clinical stability essential
- Experienced operator essential
- Experienced assistant required
- If difficulties arise and radiological screening required this is not always available.

---

in this way, the patient must be examined thoroughly and prepared for the procedure.

Preparation for percutaneous cvc insertion

Patient examination. The examination should cover the points listed in Box 6.10. The operator, wearing appropriate clothing, mask and gloves, will note the patient's anatomical landmarks, e.g. mid-sternal notch, mid third of the clavicle, external jugular vein, carotid artery, the nipple and sterno-mastoid muscle.

Box 6.10 Patient examination prior to percutaneous cvc insertion

- During examination the operator will establish the patient's understanding of the forthcoming procedure and reiterate any issues that may present themselves
- Bony landmarks and anomalies will be noted
- Centrality of the trachea will be established. Any deviation of the trachea may denote tumour, trauma possibly caused by radiotherapy, etc., and thus create potential insertion difficulties for the operator
- Patient size, height and weight noted
- Current venous access
- Venous anatomy, e.g. visual location of vessels in the neck
- Previous venous access sites, localised infection, etc.
- Obvious signs of thrombosis will be noted, e.g. dilated vessels predominantly on one side of the chest may suggest thrombosis of the great vessels of the thorax
- Swelling of the upper limbs may suggest lymphoedema or vascular occlusion of the great vessels, which could present the operator with difficulties when attempting to locate venous vessels, unless this was noted prior to the procedure
- The colour, texture and temperature of the skin will also aid the operator in the assessment and suitability of the patient condition for this type of procedure
- Chest auscultation will demonstrate to the operator the presence or absence of pleural effusion, pneumothorax and general air entry to the lungs

---

Patient preparation. Box 6.11 lists the points that should be covered in preparing the patient for percutaneous cvc insertion. Male chest hair will have been shaved prior to the procedure and any skin and hair debris removed (see Ch. 5). The chosen site of access, i.e. neck, mid-sternal notch, axilla and the arm to nipple level, should be meticulously cleaned with an alcoholic cleansing solution.

Administration of local anaesthetic. Suggestions for the safe administration of the local sedative agent are given in Box 6.12. Once the cleansing agent has been applied and the skin has dried, local anaesthetic lignocaine 1% is administered intradermally at the lower edge of the clavicle, advancing subcutaneously on an ipsilateral route for approximately 3–4 inches. This facilitates local anaesthesia for the creation of the subcutaneous tunnel in which the tunnelled catheter will eventually lie.

Adequate anaesthetic filtration will also be required for the final fixation sutures around the catheter at the point at which the catheter will exit. Local anaesthetic will also be required posteriorly to the clavicle, advancing medially and ensuring a minimum of discomfort to the patient when the rigid introducer is finally advanced into the subclavian vein. Slow injection of local anaesthetic will cause less discomfort to the patient during this stage of the procedure.

Box 6.11   Patient preparation for percutaneous cvc insertion

- The patient's haematological status will be known to the operator prior to the procedure
- The patient's consent will be obtained prior to procedure
- Male chest hair will be shaved prior to the procedure in order to reduce discomfort when dressings are replaced
- The patient will be in the supine position in a clean quiet area of the ward with good lighting and access to emergency equipment should the need arise
- The bed will be checked to ensure that all mechanisms are in a safe working order
- Emergency equipment will be checked prior to the commencement of the procedure
- A pulse oximeter will be attached to the patient's finger or toe and a baseline assessment will be made prior to sedation being administered. The oxygen saturation will be monitored continuously throughout the procedure
- A rolled towel placed between the patient's shoulders may aid the operator during the cvc insertion. This technique increases the space between the first rib and the clavicle and also aids in accentuating the landmarks of the patient's thorax and neck
- The patient will be reassured of the Trendelenburg position (see Fig. 5.1) that will be adopted for the duration of the procedure and will be positioned in a 20°, head-down position, i.e. head below the pelvis, to enable the great vessels of the thorax to become engorged with blood, making cannulation of the selected vessel straightforward
- Peripheral venous access will have been checked for patency
- Appropriate sedation will have been prescribed, diluted and prepared for administration. The appropriate reversal agent will be readily available
- The patient will be informed about each stage of the forthcoming procedure

---

Box 6.12   Suggestions for safe administration of the sedative agent to be used in the insertion of a cvc

- Ensure the patient is comfortable and in the correct position, with the selected side of the body close to the edge of the bed before sedation is administered
- Check prescription of sedative agent
- Ensure reversal agent for the sedative is immediately available
- Dilution of sedative agent will aid in small incremental doses being administered safely
- Patent, peripheral venous access is mandatory prior to the insertion of a cvc, should emergency venous access be required.
- Ensure peripheral venous access is patent by flushing with sodium chloride
- Ensure patient's clinical state is stable, e.g. blood pressure, pulse, respiratory function and oximetry are within normal limits prior to the procedure
- Inform patient that many sedatives administered intravenously may cause irritation to the vein and sting during administration. Slow administration will reduce any potential discomfort
- Once patency of peripheral venous access is established, a small test dose of sedation may be given and the effect assessed
- Continuous monitoring of the patient's oxygenation and cardiovascular system will alert the assistant to commence oxygen therapy. Oxygen saturation should ideally be maintained above 95%, unless respiratory function is impaired prior to the procedure, when oxygen should be commenced prior to commencement. Severe hypoxia, e.g. of less than 90%, should alert the operator to question whether central venous access using a subclavian approach is appropriate
- Adequate sedation should be achieved by small incremental doses prior to the operator commencing the procedure, thereby enhancing the patient's relaxation and reducing the fear so often associated with this type of cvc insertion
- The administration of any sedative must be given with great caution with consideration to the patient's size, clinical condition and previous experience of other sedative agents
- Wherever possible the patient's request to achieve an appropriate level of sedation should be respected. However, every effort should also be made to remind the patient of the effect of modern sedatives, and in particular the amnesic effect that many of these products possess

---

Insertion

Following the administration of local anaesthetic, the patient will be draped in sterile towels, ensuring that the appropriate anatomical landmarks remain clearly visible. Once the skin is prepared and local anaesthetic infiltrated, the operator may choose to change gloves, using a new and sterile pair for the insertion of the cvc. This reduces the risk of infection.

A small incision (1–3 cm) will be made approximately 2 cm below the mid third of the clavicle. Using a scalpel, fascia will be divided at this point, to allow ease of entry of the rigid introducer and splittable sheath at a later stage.

A syringe containing sodium chloride with an appropriate sized cannulation needle, often a 16 or 18 gauge, is advanced just below the mid-point of the clavicle. The syringe and needle are carefully redirected towards the mid-sternal notch. The syringe and needle will be advanced behind the clavicle parallel to the pathway of the subclavian vein. A slight negative pressure in the syringe is required until the subclavian vein is cannulated and a flashback of venous blood is seen in the syringe. Care must be taken by the operator to recognise venous blood as opposed to arterial, particularly in those patients who have cardiac symptoms or respiratory disabilities.

The syringe will be removed, leaving the needle in position within the vein. The Seldinger guidewire will initially be straightened and positioned within the needle and gently advanced into the superior vena cava. No resistance should be experienced during the advancement of the guidewire and it is vital that no effort should be exerted. Forcing of the wire may result in venous or cardiac rupture.

The guidewire must be clearly visible and held firmly in place throughout every stage of the procedure. The Seldinger wire will be left in the venous system during the creation of the subcutaneous tunnel.

Priming of the catheter. To reduce the risk of air entering the vascular system, the catheter will be primed with sodium chloride or heparinised saline prior to insertion.

Creation of the subcutaneous tunnel. The subcutaneous tunnel should travel a minimum of 3 inches below the site of cannulation on the chest wall and will be created with the use of a tunnelling rod made of either metal or plastic.

In the creation of the subcutaneous tunnel, care must be taken to maintain a superficial approach when advancing the catheter and the Dacron cuff along the subcutaneous tunnel. The Dacron cuff attached to the catheter will act as a securing mechanism, fibrosing with subcutaneous tissue over a period of time, thus preventing the catheter from falling out (Fig. 6.6).

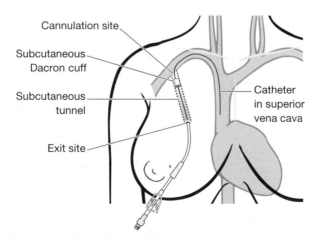

Fig. 6.6   Subcutaneous tunnel and cuff.

Extensive damage may be caused to the surrounding tissue when creating the subcutaneous tunnel unless a single approach is used, which reduces the risk of muscle damage, haematoma, infection and pain. The subcutaneous tunnel may be created either using a reverse tunnelling technique, e.g. commencing from the clavicular incision, or from the lower end of the tunnel, pulling the catheter from the nipple end up towards the patient's shoulder. The tunnelling technique will depend on the type of device used and the manufacturer's recommended technique. The second method is described below.

At the point of entry of the tunnelling rod, the patient's skin will be covered with sterile gauze, thus protecting the catheter from contact with the patient's skin. The catheter, attached to the tunnelling rod, will be pulled upwards, under the skin on the chest wall, with the Dacron cuff positioned midway along the subcutaneous tunnel, finally exiting at the original cannulation point below the clavicle.

A cuff left too close to the exit site may not always fibrose adequately and therefore there is a risk that the catheter may fall out once the sutures are removed. Care must be taken by the operator not to contaminate the catheter at this point and therefore the catheter should be handled with gauze or forceps in order to maintain a totally aseptic technique.

The tunnelling rod will be removed and, using an aseptic technique, the catheter will be cut and assessed by the operator for the final and optimal position, i.e. at the junction of the superior vena cava and right atrium. This will normally be assessed by measuring two intercostal spaces from the clavicle. X-ray screening facilities, if available, will enable the operator or radiologist to make precise decisions as to the length and position of the catheter within the vascular system.

In addition, an experienced operator will also take into account the patient's height and general shape; this allows accurate positioning to take place. For example the weight of female breast tissue may pull the catheter back, down the subcutaneous tunnel and out of position into the innominate or subclavian vein, thus increasing the risk of thrombosis or blockage.

During the next stage of the procedure where catheter access to the vein is created, the catheter should be protected from risk of contamination, in particular by contact with the patient's skin, by using a sterile drape or sterile gauze.

Introducing the catheter into the vascular system. The rigid introducer and splittable sheath will be advanced over the Seldinger wire into the subclavian vein. Both the Seldinger wire and rigid introducer will be removed, leaving the splittable sheath in position, providing access for the catheter to enter the subclavian vein. The operator will prevent air entering the vascular system by placing a thumb over the end of the splittable sheath. Using forceps, the operator will advance the tip of the catheter into the splittable sheath, peeling the sheath slowly apart as the catheter is advanced into the vein, until the entire catheter is in place and the sheath split completely and removed.

Once the catheter is positioned within the vein, aspiration of the catheter lumen will provide evidence that the catheter is situated within the vein but will not define its precise position. Heparinised saline will be instilled into the lumen of the catheter by the operator to minimise the risk of blood clot formation.

The Luer connection of the catheter will be closed by the use of a hub. Many centres find the 'closed system' method particularly useful when PN is to be administered, reducing the risk of infection entering the vascular system.

Suturing the exit and clavicular sites. On completion of the procedure skin sutures or steristrips will be applied to the clavicular site. The catheter will be secured with sutures that remain in situ until the Dacron cuff has firmly and reliably fibrosed; this usually takes about 3 weeks (see Fig. 6.7). It is essential that fibrosis is guaranteed, otherwise the catheter will fall out once these sutures are removed.

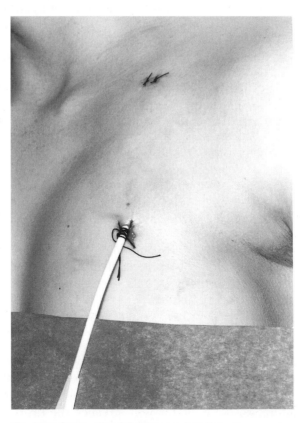

Fig. 6.7 Suture sites following cvc insertion.

Patients receiving steroid treatment will have prolonged healing powers due to their treatment and therefore additional time may be required to ensure adequate fibrosis occurring.

Post procedural observations

The patient's colour, perfusion and respiratory function must be continuously monitored by the assistant during the procedure, and the operator informed promptly of any change in the patient's comfort or condition.

Oxygen therapy may be required should the administered sedative result in respiratory depression, identified by oxygen saturation falling below 95%. Care must be taken during the procedure to note the patient's cardiac rhythm, and the operator should be notified immediately should arrhythmias be observed.

Should arrhythmias occur at this point, insertion of the Seldinger wire may have caused irritation to the electrical pathway of the heart. Gentle and minimal withdrawal of the Seldinger wire by the operator may resolve the arrhythmia. However, if this condition persists, total removal of the wire may be necessary with a full electrocardiogram performed to demonstrate the cause of the abnormal rhythm.

Reassurance of the patient by the nurse will often aid in maintaining stable vital signs during the procedure and will be much appreciated by most patients. There is much to be said in achieving adequate sedative levels but also having a patient who is able to cooperate in terms of position, etc.

Respiratory function. Monitoring of the respiratory system quarter hourly in the first hour post insertion and thereafter 4 hourly is essential and should be continued for at least 24 h post procedure.

Accurate and regular observations of the patient's respiratory function is often one of the most important observations following the insertion of a cvc. An altered respiratory pattern often provides a reliable indicator to a patient's changing physiological state. Pre-procedural parameters will be a useful guide to the patient's normal respiratory function and pattern.

The patient's conscious state should also be monitored with care following the administration of sedative agents. Many sedative agents can produce a delayed action when used in the elderly, resulting in respiratory depression and hypoxia. If sedation is thought to be the cause of an unrousable patient post sedation administered during a cvc insertion, accompanied with depressed respiratory function, the medical team may feel a reversal agent is appropriate. The effect of a reversal agent will neurologically rouse the patient and stimulate respiratory function. However, the reversal agent may only be effective in the short term. Some sedatives possess a prolonged half-life and patients experiencing symptoms of respiratory depression must be observed and monitored with care in case the action of the sedative recurs, presenting symptoms described above.

It is advisable to maintain oximetry for this purpose and administer appropriate oxygen therapy accordingly.

Baseline respiratory function and pattern will enable the medical and nursing team to detect any variance in the patient's respiratory state, highlighting early signs of possible pneumothorax or haemothorax. Symptoms of shoulder tip pain, a dry cough or back pain can all be significant following cvc insertion and may indicate the presence of a pneumothorax up to 24 h and beyond post insertion.

Cardiovascular system. Monitoring of the cardiovascular system half hourly over the first 2 h and thereafter 4 hourly is important and the relevance of anomalies must be established promptly.

Many elderly patients may be hypotensive post cvc insertion following the administration of intravenous sedation or general anaesthetic. As with all surgical procedures, the cause for hypotension should be sought.

If sedation is thought to be the cause of hypotension, the medical team may feel a reversal agent is appropriate thus neurologically rousing the patient and raising the blood pressure to within normal limits.

Symptoms of persistent tachycardia post cvc insertion should be assumed to be a result of bleeding until proven otherwise. Puncture of the arterial system can occur and may result in brisk blood loss if no action is taken. Haemorrhage is less likely to occur in the hands of an experienced operator. However, damage to small vessels, both arterial and venous, of which the operator may be unaware, may occur during the fashioning of the subcutaneous tunnel. On occasion these vessels may ooze excessively, particularly in patients with haematological diseases. A pressure dressing added to the original dressing will aid clot formation and often stem this oozing. However, if this continues over a period of hours or days it may be necessary for a surgical approach to be taken.

In the event that the procedure may have been particularly traumatic, perhaps with considerable blood loss resulting in a reduced circulating blood volume, replacement fluids or blood products may be indicated in the resuscitation of the patient's cardiovascular state to normal limits.

Suggestions for controlling bleeding are discussed in Chapter 10.

Arrhythmias. Previous cardiac arrhythmias noted prior to the insertion of the cvc should be available for comparison in the event that further arrhythmias present during or post cvc insertion.

Spontaneous ventricular ectopics or supraventricular tachycardia during or post insertion of a cvc may be explained if the tip of the cvc is situated in the right ventricle. This may cause irritation to the myocardium and the electrical pathway of the heart, resulting in an arrhythmia.

Following confirmation of the catheter position by chest X-ray, the tip of the catheter may be slightly too far advanced within the superior vena cava and the catheter may need to be withdrawn slightly, reducing the risk of cardiac arrhythmias. A repeat chest X-ray will confirm the correct

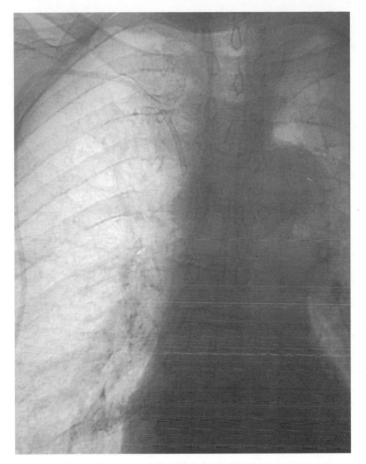

Fig. 6.8 Chest X-ray demonstrating cvc position.

positioning of the cvc (Fig. 6.8). The symptoms of an arrhythmia will often resolve once correct placement is assured.

In the unusual event that a cvc may be required in patients with trans-venous pacing wires, only the most experienced operators should attempt this procedure.

Pain. Cvc insertion is often described as uncomfortable, usually as a result of the necessary position, but it is rarely painful in the hands of an experienced operator who uses adequate quantities of local anaesthetic and sedation.

Discomfort often presents 3–4 h post insertion and can be relieved by mild analgesia. However, pain associated with respiration should be promptly assessed by an experienced member of the medical team.

Shoulder tip pain around the cvc insertion site below the clavicle may be associated with trauma inflicted by the cannulation needle to the lateral pectoral nerve. Tingling of the fingers is another sign of nerve damage and may also be associated with cvc insertion. Diagnosis of nerve damage will be determined by clinical examination and not be revealed on X-ray. Urgent medical assessment to ascertain accurately the cause and true extent of pain following cvc insertion should be sought while analgesia or alternative methods of pain relief, e.g. thermal heat pad, are administered.

The most common cause of shoulder tip pain, coupled with shallow breathing, is pneumothorax. A chest X-ray will confirm this. The extent of the pneumothorax will determine the need for further intervention such as chest drainage to facilitate the extrapleural drainage of air. In some cases a patient may develop a dry irritating cough or slight pain around the affected shoulder some hours post procedure. Care must be taken not to be dismissive of these apparent minor features. A repeat chest X-ray may confirm the suspicion of a delayed pneumothorax, which may then require chest drainage. This situation is often associated with younger patients who may have a high pain threshold and assume that a certain amount of pain is normal.

General observations. Skin colour and texture is also a useful and non-invasive method of assessment in a patient who has recently undergone a procedure of this type. A cold and clammy texture to the skin may indicate shock due to sedation, excessive blood loss, or major trauma caused during the insertion of the cvc.

It can be appreciated how important accurate and regular monitoring is following cvc insertion, whether the method is surgical or percutaneous.

Complications associated with percutaneous cvc insertion

Vascular complications/catheter redirection. When using either the surgical or percutaneous subclavian approach, a cvc can occasionally pass into the jugular vein, advance distally, position in the ventricle or simply pass into the opposite subclavian vein.

Incorrect placement, particularly when the cvc is situated in the jugular vein and not repositioned, may cause cerebral thrombosis. In the majority of these situations the catheter will need replacing, but in some cases redirection may be achieved using radiological guidance. A radiologist may insert a fine wire into the catheter, redirecting it into the correct position. This can only be performed by the radiologist, using sophisticated radiological facilities.

Catheters placed in the right ventricle may cause arrhythmias, as discussed in earlier paragraphs, or may facilitate cardiac tamponade as a result of the catheter puncturing the ventricle wall. Penetration of the catheter tip through the venous wall is a rare but dangerous complication, manifesting itself once PN is commenced.

Altered respiratory pattern and dyspnoea become apparent and are precipitated either by bleeding into the mediastinum or infusion of PN directly into the mediastinum. Unless these symptoms are noted early with prompt and appropriate action taken, this situation can be a potentially fatal event.

Chest X-ray will determine the position of the catheter, whereupon a decision will be made as to the safest method of achieving correct placement. In addition to complications associated with catheter redirection, most other complications involve damage to local structures. However, an operator experienced in this procedure will reduce the incidence of redirection and pneumothorax by strict attention to precise and repetitive technique.

Haemorrhage. Arterial puncture of the carotid or subclavian arteries is a well-recognised complication and will be clearly apparent to the operator at the time of puncture. Prolonged pressure applied to the arterial vessel by the operator will normally stem excessive bleeding if normal clotting profiles have been obtained in the preparation of the patient.

It is not uncommon for a large haematoma to develop following arterial puncture. Placing the patient in a 45° upright position, with a pressure bandage over the area, will aid drainage of the haematoma and encourage haemostasis to occur. In more severe cases of arterial puncture, when symptoms may include hypotension, tachycardia, sweating and a feeling of faintness, urgent surgical intervention may be required.

Haemorrhage is less likely to occur in the hands of an experienced operator, owing to his knowledge of vascular anatomy and experience in cannulating the great vessels of the neck and thorax. However, during the creation of the subcutaneous tunnel some invisible vessels may be damaged, causing both the clavicular and the exit site of the subcutaneous tunnel to ooze excessively. A pressure dressing will often stem this oozing, but if this continues over a period of time it may be necessary for a more surgical approach to be taken. In many cases a pressure dressing placed over the initial dressing may assist in encouraging fibrin to form around the bleeding point.

In the haematological group of patients who are dependent on blood products, urgent assessment and replacement of these products must be sought. Haemostasis may be achieved by either the use of a haemostatic agent placed topically or alternatively a ligature or diathermy to the bleeding site may be considered.

Pneumothorax. The hazard of pneumothorax complicating subclavian catheterisation is the most well known and obvious risk. Pneumothorax (air in the pleural space) will be identified on chest X-ray and diagnosed by the radiologist, who will then advise on intervention if necessary.

In the case of pneumothorax the patient may complain of chest pain and dyspnoea. Clinically, there is hyperesonance to percussion and an absence of breath sounds over the affected side of the chest. The chest X-

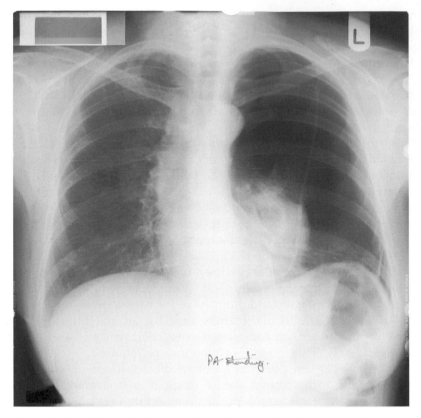

Fig. 6.9 Chest X-ray of left pneumothorax demonstrating the absence of lung markings, with the lung appearing shrunken above the left diaphragm.

ray will highlight the absence of lung markings, with the lung appearing shrunken and visible at the hilum on X-ray (Fig. 6.9).

The insertion of a chest drain, to relieve the patient's symptoms and to reinflate the lung, will generally only be necessary if the pneumothorax exceeds 20%. Smaller pneumothoraces are more difficult to diagnose on chest X-ray with a slightly discernible lung edge away from the chest wall. Clinically the patient with a small pneumothorax may be asymptomatic, lacking shoulder tip or general chest pain that may be associated with pneumothorax. This situation will often not require intervention, but close monitoring of respiratory symptoms and repeated chest X-ray to evaluate the reinflation of the affected lung.

The question of delayed pneumothorax has also been discussed, where a slow pleural leak only presents over a period of hours, despite an apparent normal chest X-ray post insertion.

Haemothorax. In the case of haemothorax, air and blood will accumulate in the pleural space, resulting from the puncture of both a blood vessel and the pleura during central venous cannulation. In this situation, respiratory function may be severely compromised with a brisk deterioration in the patient's general condition.

Small amounts of blood in the pleural space will not require drainage and usually resolve satisfactorily. However, larger losses will require formal drainage using underwater seal drainage, allowing accurate assessment of blood loss and reinflation of the lung.

Air embolism. Embolism may be avoided by utilising the head-down (Trendelenburg, see Fig. 5.1) position. Care must be taken by the operator when preparing to insert the catheter. This is done by priming the catheter with sodium chloride or heparinised saline, which reduces the risk of air entering the venous circulation.

Neurological damage. Neurological damage to the brachial plexus may also be a result of cannulation. Symptoms of tingling of the face and fingers may be symptomatic of brachial plexus damage. Many of these complications will rarely be seen in the hands of an experienced operator.

Cardiac tamponade. This complication is extremely rare, particularly in the hands of one experienced in the procedure of central venous cannulation. This situation can be avoided by the use of a J-tipped Seldinger wire which is soft and pliable and avoids the risk of puncturing cardiac muscle.

Infection. This complication is well recognised in the administration of therapies via the central venous route; it is discussed extensively in Chapters 1 and 7.

A peripheral approach to central venous cannulation

This type of central venous access may be an ideal alternative for those patients who are unsuitable for infraclavicular placement of a tunnelled cvc owing to thrombosis, respiratory distress, infection, anatomical anomalies, and for those who are unable to receive sedative medications because of their clinical condition.

Patient assessment is essential in both methods of insertion; however, for peripheral insertion accurate patient examination and specific assessment of the venous anatomy of the arm is mandatory. PICC catheters are suitable for both long-term and short-term episodes of PN, although unless clinically necessary a PICC catheter is usually used for the patient requiring short- to medium-term PN.

Patient examination

The specific features of patient examination prior to PICC insertion are listed in Box 6.13.

Box 6.13 Patient examination prior to PICC insertion

- Examination of the patient's skeletal system, noting any anatomical anomalies, arthritis, or obvious clavicular fractures, will often highlight potential difficulties in catheter advancement
- During examination the patient will be assessed for signs of thrombosis, lymphoedema, etc.
- Infection associated with previous peripheral venous sites will be avoided by selecting the opposite arm
- Detailed examination of the venous system within the arm will be assessed by the operator
- Appropriate venous site selected
- The approximate distance from antecubital fossa to the superior vena cava (svc) will be measured by the operator to determine accurate positioning of the PICC within the svc
- The patient's mobility will also be assessed at this stage. PICCs are not advisable in patients who require wheelchairs or crutches, owing to the risk of phlebitis caused by friction of the catheter within the vein

---

Patient preparation

The same attention must be paid to the preparation of a patient receiving a PICC as described for percutaneous cvc insertion (see Boxes 6.14, 6.15).

Immediately prior to catheter insertion the local anaesthetic cream applied earlier to the patient's arm will be removed by the assistant. The patient's arm will be thoroughly cleansed with an alcoholic solution and allowed to dry completely. Maki et al (1991) recommend the use of chlorhexidine as a cleansing agent, providing the solution is allowed to dry

---

Box 6.14 Essential requirements for PICC insertion

- The procedure will take place in a quiet and clean area of the ward
- The bed mechanics will be checked and ensured to be functional
- Good lighting will be available
- The patient will be positioned in a comfortable position in bed with the selected arm extended at a 90° angle on a pillow on a bed table

---

Box 6.15 Patient preparation

- Patient information
- Patient consent
- Recent clotting profile and platelet count above 60
- Precise examination of venous access in antecubital fossa, e.g. basilic, cephalic and median cubital veins
- Forearm hair shaved
- Patient positioned in upright position in bed, with selected arm extended at a 90° angle on bed table
- Local anaesthetic cream applied to antecubital fossa over proposed site of access 1 h prior to the procedure

completely. The assistant will apply a tourniquet to the patient's upper arm, encouraging filling of the larger vessels in the arm. The selected area will be draped in sterile towels once the skin is dry.

Insertion of a PICC

There are several different designs of PICC. Some have a Seldinger wire design, while others incorporate a stiffened plastic material or a splittable sheath (see Figs 4.4, 4.5). However, the principles of insertion remain similar.

The catheter is primed with sodium chloride to limit the risk of air entering the venous system. The operator will introduce the cannula into the selected vein until flashback of blood is seen in the cannulation device. The assistant will then release the tourniquet. The operator will remove the needle section of the cannulation device, leaving the cannula in the vein. Using an aseptic, non-touch technique the operator will advance the catheter into the venous circulation, via the cannula.

No pressure or effort should be exerted to advance the catheter at any stage. If insertion is successful and no obstruction is apparent, the patient should turn her head towards the operator, placing the chin on the chest, thus preventing the catheter from advancing into the vessels of the neck. The operator will recall the measurement made earlier and position the catheter at the approximate point of the superior vena cava, which will later be determined by chest X-ray.

If the Seldinger wire method is used the wire will be removed at this stage, followed by the venous cannula, leaving the catheter positioned in the vein. In the case of the splittable sheath method the catheter will be advanced into the vein and, once the desired length is inserted, the sheath will split, leaving the catheter positioned within the vein. Luer housing will be applied to the distal end of the catheter, whereupon aspiration will determine venous position. However, chest X-ray is essential to determine the ultimate and correct position of the PICC (Fig. 6.10).

At the securing stage of the procedure care should be taken to limit the movement of the catheter as this will reduce the risk of phlebitis. Once meticulously clean and dry, steristrips may be applied to the site to ensure stability. A non-adhesive dressing may then be applied and a waterproof dressing to offer additional stability. The waterproof dressing, extended to incorporate the PICC external to the skin, placed on the forearm, will also aid in the general stability of the device and will help to reduce mechanical phlebitis (Figs 6.10, 6.11). Suturing of the catheter to the skin may also be an option. However, care should be taken not to puncture the PICC during suturing. A length of elasticated bandage applied to the arm will also provide support and protection for the PICC catheter.

Despite the ease of insertion of this type of cvc in comparison to a

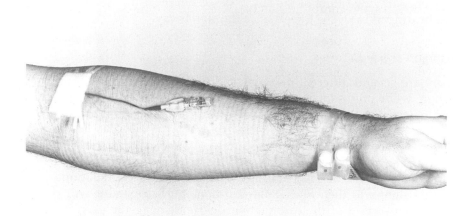

Fig. 6.10   PICC line positioned within the median cubital vein.

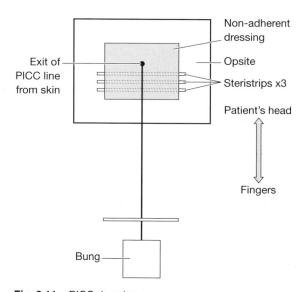

Fig. 6.11   PICC dressing.

percutaneous, subclavian approach, it is imperative to remember that the tip of this device is in the same position as that of the infraclavicularly inserted device described earlier. For this reason it must attract the same degree of detailed and meticulous care. Chest X-ray will be required to determine the position of this catheter prior to its use.

Postprocedural observations and complications of PICCs

The most common complication in the use of this type of device is oozing from the site of venepuncture. This is related to the recommended platelet count prior to the procedure. As with percutaneous cvc insertion, it is advisable to apply pressure but not disturb the original dressing.

Owing to the absence of sedative requirement for the insertion of a cvc of this type, it would be unusual for patients to develop respiratory complications following this type of procedure. The incidence of cardiovascular complications is also reduced, but the position of the tip of the catheter is important and can still present arrhythmias if advanced too far into the cardiac system.

The main issue concerning this type of device is the risk of contamination in the insertion and subsequent management. Phlebitis can present real problems, normally associated with women whose veins are too small for the selected device, resulting in friction within the vein. Heat administered via a pad or covered hot water bottle will dilate the vessel and often reduce the friction action. Glyceryl trinitrate patches have also been shown to relieve these symptoms (Richardson & Bruso 1993, Gabriel 1996, Oakley 1997).

AVOIDING COMPLICATIONS IN THE USE OF CVCS USED FOR PN

Avoiding complications in the use of cvcs for PN may be accomplished by setting a strict protocol, covering every aspect in the preparation of the patient, examination, monitoring and long-term management of the cvc. Meticulous attention to the aseptic technique and general management of the PN catheter will ensure a trouble-free episode of artificial nutrition for the patient.

An operator experienced in this procedure is also essential if the complications associated with this high-risk procedure are to be limited. If this strict and disciplined approach is not adopted and enforced, then infection of the cvc will be inevitable.

DISCUSSION

Central venous catheters used for the administration of PN, although associated with recognised complications, are a satisfactory means to provide nutritional support to a specific group of patients. The success in the performance of cvcs depends on detailed and accurate patient assessment in order that the correct and most appropriate device is selected for the compromised patient. This chapter has discussed how, having achieved this assessment, it is possible to decide the method by which the catheter is to be inserted.

The method of insertion will depend on the patient's clinical condition. Much of the information required to assess this is provided by the ward nursing team. This information will guide the operator to insert a suitable central venous access device with the minimum distress to the patient. Guarantee of these factors will increase the likelihood of successful insertion and subsequent management of the cvc used for PN.

It is the operator who holds the primary responsibility for the aseptic technique, including scrupulous handwashing, necessary to ensure minimum risk of catheter-related sepsis during the insertion of a cvc. However, it is the ward nurse who, familiar with the patient's fears and anxieties, will reassure, support and assist in the insertion of the device to be used for PN.

Despite modern advances in catheter design and the development of new and improved materials, complications associated with central venous cannulation will only be minimised if total commitment is afforded to the monitoring and close observation of the patient post catheter insertion.

The performance of the cvc in PN is an essential aspect of this therapy. Successful administration of vital nutrients can only be achieved if reliable central venous access is available and precise aseptic management is assured.

REFERENCES

Bo-Linn G, Anderson D, Anderson K, McGoon M, Osler Medical House Staff 1982 Percutaneous central venous catheterization performed by medical house officers: a prospective study. Catheterization and Cardiovascular Diagnosis 8:23.
Editorial 1986 Central venous catheterisation. Lancet 2:669
Elliott T, Farouqi M, Armstrong R et al 1994 Guidelines for good practice in central venous cannulation. Journal of Hospital Infection 28:163–176
Freedmans E, Bosserman G 1993 Tunnelled catheters. Nursing Clinics of North America 28(4):851–858
Gabriel J 1996 Care and management of peripherally inserted central catheters. British Journal of Nursing, Surgical Nurse 5(10):594–599
Hamilton H, Fermo K 1998 Assessment of patients requiring I.V. therapy via a central venous route. British Journal of Nursing 7(8):451–460
Maki D, Ringer M, Alvardo C 1991 Prospective randomised trial of povidone iodine, alcohol and chlorhexadine for prevention of infections associated with central venous and arterial catheters. Lancet 338:339–343
Oakley C 1997 Peripherally inserted central venous catheters: the experience of a specialist oncology department. Journal of Cancer Nursing 1(1):50–53
Richardson D, Bruso P 1993 Vascular access devices: management of common complications. Journal of Intravenous Nursing 16(1):44–49
Sznajder J, Zveibil F, Bitterman H, Weiner P, Bursztein S 1986 Central venous catheterization: failure and complication rates by three percutaneous approaches. Archives of Internal Medicine 146:259
Traeger SM, Williams GB, Milliren G 1986 Total parenteral nutrition by a Nutrition Support Team: improved quality of care. Journal of Parenteral and Enteral Nutrition 10:408–412

FURTHER READING

East S 1994 Planning, implementation and evaluation of a successful hospital based peripheral inserted central catheter program. Journal of Intravenous Nursing 17(4):189–192

Gilston A 1976 Cannulation of the femoral vessel. British Journal of Anaesthesia 48:500

Goodwin M 1993 The percutaneously inserted central catheter. Journal of Intravenous Nursing 16(2):92–100

Horden J, Kemp L, Mirtallo J 1995 Femoral catheters increase risk of infection in Total Parenteral Nutrition patients. Nutrition, Clinical Practice 10: 60–66.

Moncrief J 1958 Femoral catheters. Annals of Surgery 147:166

Purdue G, Hunt J 1986 Vascular access through a femoral vessel: indications and complications. Journal of Burn Care and Rehabilitation 7:498–500

7

Nursing management

Jan Tait

Introduction
Introducing the patient and his family to PN
Assessment of the patient prior to the commencement of PN

Monitoring the patient on PN
Complications associated with PN
Other nursing issues
Guidelines and policies for catheter management

INTRODUCTION

This chapter addresses the issues of the management of patients receiving parenteral nutrition (PN). It also introduces the generic issues relating to the nursing management of a central venous catheter (cvc) and the importance of management in relation to PN.

The use of nutritional support has increased in recent years and therefore it is likely that many nurses responsible for the care of the malnourished patient will encounter the use of PN. In some hospitals the management of these patients is the responsibility of a Nutrition Support Team (NST), Nutrition Support Committee (NSC), or nutrition nurse specialist. However, in many other hospitals without access to a NST, the responsibility for the safe administration of PN falls to the ward nurse.

Unfortunately, the administration of artificial nutrition has profound physiological and metabolic effects. Any technique involving the insertion of a cvc, creation of a subcutaneous tunnel, plus the intravenous administration of complex solutions, cannot be without hazards. The use of PN is associated with life-threatening complications, particularly infection (Sitges-Serra et al 1995). However, these complications can be significantly reduced if staff are educated in the safe administration and management of PN (Mughal 1989).

This chapter is aimed at the ward nurse and provides information that will increase the nurse's knowledge and confidence in caring for the patient receiving PN. It cannot be stressed sufficiently that staff involved in the administration of PN must follow research-based protocols to reduce the risk of serious complications occurring to the compromised patient.

Nursing staff have a particularly prominent role in the care of the catheter and administration of PN. However, for many nurses these issues may not have been covered in their pre-registration training. *The Scope of Professional Practice* (UKCC 1992b) states that the registered nurse must 'honestly acknowledge any limits of personal knowledge and skill and take steps to remedy any relevant deficits in order effectively and appropriately to meet the needs of patients and clients'. The care of the PN catheter is undoubtedly safer in the hands of nursing staff experienced in cvc management. In the past it has often been easier for the nurse to refuse to accept responsibility for the tasks and shift the responsibility to medical staff. However, the modern nurse should consider the *Code of Professional Practice* (UKCC 1992a), which states that the registered nurse must 'safeguard and promote the interests and well-being of patients and clients'. The combination of complex nutrients delivered via the parenteral route can have disastrous consequences unless great respect is afforded to this therapy. It is the ward nurse who will be instrumental in the safe administration and monitoring of the catheter used for PN.

A structured teaching package is useful and should be available for all nurses responsible for the care of a patient receiving PN. This should include information that encompasses both theory and practice. Box 7.1 lists objectives that should be covered.

INTRODUCING THE PATIENT AND HIS FAMILY TO PN

Prior to the commencement of treatment, it is essential to provide the patient and his family with information regarding PN. Patients requiring PN following a period of malnutrition are, by definition, often seriously ill. The inability to eat may have a demoralising effect, and the introduction of nutritional support will often be greeted with relief both by the patient and his family.

The importance and relevance of artificial nutrition plus the need for constant monitoring should be discussed. The issue of artificial nutrition and the method by which it is to be delivered may be alarming for many patients and their families; simple explanation and reassurance by the nursing team throughout the treatment period is therefore essential. The

---

Box 7.1   Learning objectives for care of a patient receiving PN

The nurse should be able to:

- Discuss the indications for PN
- Describe the advantages and disadvantages of central and peripheral catheters
- Describe the variable types of catheters available and their indications for use
- Describe the potential complications associated with the insertion of a cvc
- Discuss how microorganisms can be transmitted into the vascular system
- Demonstrate an ability to perform effective handwashing technique
- Discuss measures taken to avoid catheter-related sepsis
- Describe the metabolic complications associated with the administration of PN
- Describe other complications associated with PN therapy
- Demonstrate an ability to operate infusion pumps and to detect and solve problems associated with the pumps
- Demonstrate an ability to carry out procedures efficiently and safely

nurse will provide vital support and encouragement for the malnourished patient who will, in the early stages of treatment, often appear demoralised, lack confidence and have little interest in events occurring around him.

If at this stage long-term nutritional support is being considered, it is essential that the patient and his family are kept fully informed of the anticipated duration and the major implications for a change in their lifestyle, particularly if home PN (HPN) is envisaged.

If the patient had been chronically unwell and has been suffering from malnutrition for some time the information and support may be quite different. Malnutrition often affects the patient's physical appearance as well as his psychological state, with symptoms of depression being quite common. It is important that the patient and his family are able to understand the effects that adequate nutrition can have on a person and the potential benefit of this treatment.

ASSESSMENT OF THE PATIENT PRIOR TO THE COMMENCEMENT OF PN

Patient selection should be carried out by a multidisciplinary team. There are several factors that should be taken into account before treatment with PN is established. It is not appropriate for all patients to receive nutritional support in the form of PN, as the treatment can be associated with complications that may be avoided by using alternative methods. The following questions will aid the nurse in identifying the malnourished patient who will benefit from PN.

- Does the patient have a functioning gastrointestinal (GI) tract?
- Is the patient at risk from further malnutrition?
- Will the patient benefit from PN?
- Can the patient's nutritional needs be met with enteral nutrition?
- Is PN the most appropriate method of providing nutrition to the malnourished patient?

A thorough assessment by the NST is necessary before PN treatment can be commenced. Detailed assessment of the patient's clinical condition is required prior to insertion of the cvc; this is described fully in Chapter 6. In addition to preparing the patient for catheter insertion, the NST will also require detailed clinical and biochemical assessment to ensure the patient will benefit from PN.

Baseline measurements

Before treatment commences it is important to establish baseline measurements. Blood pressure, temperature, pulse and respiration should be documented. The patient's height, weight and body mass index (BMI) should be recorded on admission, as well as a record of normal dietary intake, any signs and symptoms that may have affected intake, or gastrointestinal disturbances such as diarrhoea or vomiting. Biochemical measurements should be documented and correction of electrolytes, hydration, coagulopathy and sepsis addressed to ensure maximum stability prior to the commencement of PN.

Calculation of nutritional requirements

A dietitian will calculate the patient's nutritional requirements. It is important to note that this assessment is an estimate and may need adjustment, depending on the individual patient's daily nutritional and fluid requirements. This calculation should take into account the patient's height, weight, mobility and septic status (see Ch. 8). Consideration should also be given to the patient's underlying medical condition and current clinical condition, which may influence the overall volume of fluid and the rate at which PN is administered. For example, a malnourished, oedematous patient will probably require a reduced volume of fluid in the form of PN, or the same volume of fluid infused over a longer period of time. This will reduce the risk of fluid overload and aid in the limitation of oedema.

Nutritional requirements may need to be increased when the patient is septic or stressed, for example following major surgery. Fluid losses sustained via a fistula may also influence the patient's electrolyte and fluid requirements on a daily basis.

During the dietetic assessment of the patient, anthropometric measurements (skinfold thickness) are often used to indicate to the NST the degree of malnutrition the patient is experiencing. Combined with clinical assessment, this will provide the dietitian with valuable information regarding the patient's nutritional requirements.

MONITORING THE PATIENT ON PN

Monitoring the patient who is receiving PN is one of the most vital aspects of care contributing to a successful outcome of therapy. Careful monitoring allows the clinician to:

- ensure that the nutritional needs of the patient are being met
- assess the effectiveness of treatment
- allow for the early detection of complications.

The nurse has a particularly important role in the management and monitoring of the patient receiving PN. The nursing staff directly responsible for the management of the patient should have the ability to recognise important changes in the patient's condition. The nurse should therefore be constantly alert for the development of complications, both metabolic and mechanical. Symptoms often apparently unrelated to the administration of PN are regularly assessed by the nurse. For example, a change in respiratory patterns, peripheral oedema, or sudden fevers are all subtle symptoms that may be relevant to complications associated with PN. Prompt recognition of changes in the patient's general condition can alert and guide the clinician to carry out further investigation and clinical assessment.

The use of a protocol provides a structure and guidance to the less experienced clinician and nurse, and will aid in the prompt recognition and reduction of metabolic complications (Anderson et al 1996). Daily monitoring of weight, fluid balance, blood glucose and urinalysis are all invaluable nursing observations that will guide the NST in prescribing the correct volume of nutritional fluid for the patient with intestinal failure. Regular monitoring of biochemical measurements will detect metabolic complications promptly and is essential in the safe administration of complex nutrients via the venous system.

Careful observation and clinical assessment can often highlight potential complications at an early stage. The frequency of monitoring will depend upon the stage of treatment the patient is in and will often be dependent on the patient's underlying condition, for example small bowel fistulae resulting in excessive fluid and electrolyte losses.

Monitoring of the PN patient is discussed in detail below, separated into clinical observation and laboratory monitoring.

Clinical observation

This section will address the importance of routine observations made by the nurse and focus on the relevance of these to PN

Vital signs

The regular monitoring of vital signs is particularly important following central catheter insertion, as pneumothorax and catheter misplacement can occur even in the hands of the most experienced operator. These observations should be recorded half hourly initially, thereafter hourly recordings for the following 4–6 h should suffice.

Monitoring of respiratory and cardiovascular function post catheter insertion is of particular importance and should be performed hourly. Any alteration in respiratory function, shoulder pain or cardiac arrhythmias may have relevance to the central catheter insertion and should be reported immediately to the medical practitioner. Symptoms of a delayed or current problem are often detected following careful monitoring by the nursing staff. Complications associated with cvc insertion can manifest themselves up to 3 days post catheter insertion. For example, it may take many hours for the lung to deflate following a small accidental puncture of the lung during catheter insertion. It is only by detailed attention in monitoring the patient's vital signs that potentially life-threatening complications will be avoided.

In addition to the immediate monitoring of vital signs post central line insertion, regular 4–6 hourly monitoring of temperature, pulse and respiration is necessary to highlight the early signs of catheter-related sepsis, fluid overload, etc.

Fluid balance

An accurate record of fluid intake and output is an important piece of information that will be required by the NST before estimating the patient's nutritional and fluid requirements for the following day. It is important that the nurse has knowledge of the physiology of fluid and electrolyte balance to enable understanding of the importance of recording and maintaining an accurate fluid balance on the patient receiving PN. Symptoms are often only present in severe fluid loss or gain. It is therefore very important that the nurse has the ability to monitor and recognise the relevance of fluid status.

Fluid volume deficit (FVD) will arise when water loss exceeds water intake. The signs and symptoms of FVD are listed in Box 7.2. Fluid volume deficit can be described as:

- isotonic fluid volume deficit – equal water and sodium loss
- dehydration – loss of water exceeds sodium loss, resulting in a high sodium (hypernatraemia)
- hyponatraemic dehydration – sodium losses exceed water losses.

Fluid volume deficit can develop slowly or rapidly, the latter particularly in those patients with short gut, and the effects on the patient vary depending on the severity of the loss. It is important that the nurse is aware

---

Box 7.2   Signs and symptoms related to fluid volume deficit

- Acute weight loss
- Decreased urinary output
- Thirst/dryness of mouth
- Tongue turgor
- Skin turgor
- Pinched facial expression
- Tachycardia
- Low CVP
- Weak thready pulse
- Postural hypotension

---

of the causes of FVD and is able to identify if the patient is at particular risk of dehydration.

The causes of FVD include:

- decreased fluid intake
- polyuria
- losses of GI fluids through vomiting, diarrhoea and fistula drainage
- fever with resulting fluid loss via the skin and increased respiratory rate
- third space losses – fluid can be lost into body compartments such as the abdomen in ascites. Such losses are difficult to quantify, which is why daily weight is so important.

Normal hydration should be achieved and maintained. However, there are situations when the patient is at risk of fluid volume excess (FVE). Fluid volume excess can occur as a result of abnormal retention of water and sodium. It can be caused by a failure of the patient's regulatory systems, as in cardiac failure or renal failure. It can also occur with overzealous administration of fluids or excessive ingestion of sodium. It is essential that the nurse is able to recognise the symptoms of FVE (see Box 7.3) and alert and guide the clinician to carry out further assessment on the patient. If the patient has signs of FVE after initiation of intravenous therapy, then the rate of the infusion should be reduced.

Accurate measurement of fluid output should include urinary output and fluid losses such as diarrhoea, vomiting, fistula and gastric aspirate in addition to insensible losses. Nurses rarely consider insensible losses when recording fluid balance. However, insensible loss is an important issue for the NST when calculating the patient's individual fluid requirements in PN. Losses from respiratory exhalation and from the skin in the form of sweating over a 24 h period can amount to 800 ml, or considerably more if the patient is pyrexial or tachypnoeic. These factors should all be considered when fluid balance is calculated.

For some reason nursing staff do not always see the importance of recording fluid balance and do not treat it as a priority. Burns (1992) finds it difficult to understand why nursing staff place such importance in pulse

---

Box 7.3   Signs and symptoms of fluid volume excess

- Acute weight gain
- Breathlessness
- Filling of neck veins
- Oedema
- Puffy eyelids
- Pitting oedema
- Raised CVP
- Full bounding pulse

and respiration but do not place the same importance in recording fluid balance. It can be very helpful to enlist the help of the mobile patient in recording input and output. This often ensures the most reliable and accurate fluid balance.

Owing to the historical inaccuracy of fluid charts, it has been suggested that a more effective management of recording the patient's fluid balance may be achieved by weighing the patient daily. If changes of weight are to be measured accurately, as described below, then the weight must be measured at the same time every day. In this way the fluid balance is included in the weight measurement (Daffurn et al 1994).

Daily weight

Weight changes of more than 0.5 kg to 1 kg in a 24 h period can only be attributed to changes in fluid balance, as lean body mass cannot be accumulated that rapidly. The accuracy of weighing patients daily can vary, and will depend on what time of day the patient is weighed and whether the same scales have been used. As with other serial measurements, it is important to record the trend; this is where weight charts are particularly helpful. Methany (1996) suggests that the following practices should be carried out when recording a patient's weight:

- use the same scales
- measure weight in the morning before breakfast after voiding
- ensure the patient is in similar clothing
- use slings or underbed scales for patients who are unable to stand.

It is recommended that weight is recorded daily at the beginning of treatment to estimate fluid balance. However, this may be reduced to weekly when changes in tissue mass are observed. Body weight changes depend on the presence of fat, protein and water, and although it has limitations a steady weight gain can be indicative of a positive response to nutritional support. If the patient has been on long-term treatment it is often encouraging for him to witness an increase in weight. Therefore, the relevance of a steady weight gain should be explained to the patient and his family.

Strength

There are various ways of measuring or observing patients' strength. One of these methods is the use of a hand grip dynamometer (Fig. 7.1). The handgrip is held in the non-dominant hand and squeezed. The patient repeats this three times with the highest reading recorded. Serial measurements need to be recorded on a regular basis in order to plot the progress of the patient's strength. The nurse caring for the patient is possibly the best person, along with the patient himself, to judge strength or weakness.

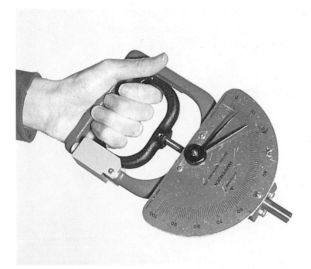

Fig. 7.1 Hand grip dynamometer.

Merely shaking hands can give the medical and nursing staff an estimate of the patient's strength. The nurse will be instrumental in monitoring the strength of a patient while assisting the patient during a bed bath or observing the patient's ability to walk increasing distances.

Anthropometric measurements

As body weight is not an accurate guide to increased body fat and muscle, which may be influenced by fluid retention, the dietitian will measure fat and skeletal muscle to monitor the effect of the nutritional support. This involves the measurement of triceps skinfold thickness and mid-arm circumference. The first is taken with the use of specially designed callipers (Fig. 7.2) and the second is measured using a tape measure. Taking anthropometric measurements is a skilled technique that can be painful if performed by inexperienced personnel. Therefore it should only be carried out by experienced dietetic staff.

General monitoring and observation

The importance of the nurse/patient relationship in observing change in nutritional status is vital. Often the nursing staff pick up the first clues that can guide the clinician to investigate nutritional status further.

- Is the patient's hair thinning?
- Is there hair loss noted on the pillow?

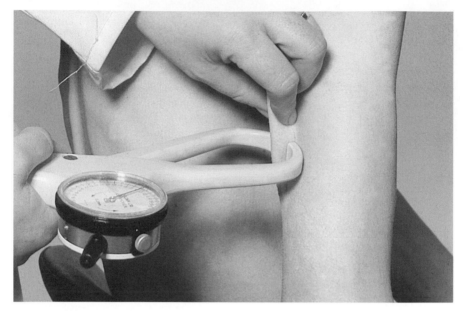

Fig. 7.2 Anthropometric callipers used by the dietitian in nutritional assessment to establish skeletal muscle mass.

- Did the family mention that the patient looks pale?
- Is there evidence of conjunctival or generalised jaundice?
- Is there evidence of skin rashes or skin irritations when bathing the patient?
- Does the patient complain of a dry mouth?

Laboratory observation

Monitoring patients receiving PN will also involve biochemical and haematological investigations.

1. Measurement of haemoglobin concentration and haematocrit in correlation with fluid balance and weight measurements can be useful when determining the fluid requirements of a patient receiving PN.
2. Routine assessment of the patient's urea and electrolyte status will aid in monitoring renal function.
3. Routine monitoring of the blood glucose level is essential to ensure that the patient is not developing hyperglycaemia due to the glucose element of the nutritional provision.
4. Monitoring and analysis of the patient's urine to detect abnormalities such as glycosuria, which may be present in the hyperglycaemic

Table 7.1 Monitoring guidelines for the patient on PN

	Start of PN	6 h following lipid infusion	Hospital PN	Home PN
Weight	√		daily	
Fluid balance			daily	
Glucose	√		daily	3-monthly
Biochemical profile	√		weekdays	3-monthly
Urea and electrolytes			weekends	
FBC	√		twice weekly	3-monthly
Magnesium	√		weekly	3-monthly
Triglycerides		√	weekly	3-monthly
Coagulation studies (INR)	√		weekly	3-monthly
Zinc, Cu			monthly	3-monthly
Zinc, Cu, Cr, manganese, selenium, red cell glutathione peroxidase			2-monthly	3-monthly
Vitamins A, C, E, B_1, B_6, B_{12}			2-monthly	
24 h urine Na, K, creatinine, urea			as indicated	as indicated

FBC, full blood count; INR, international normalised ratio.

patient, or the presence of ketones caused by a metabolic response to starvation, is essential.
5. Estimation of nitrogen balance can provide a method of determining the patient's response to nutritional support. This can be recorded by estimating the difference between nitrogen in the form of PN and the amount excreted. Nitrogen can be measured in the form of 24 h urine collections, fistulae output and blood tests.

The frequency of monitoring biochemistry and haematology will often depend on the patient's clinical condition. Table 7.1 provides guidelines for monitoring the patient receiving PN.

COMPLICATIONS ASSOCIATED WITH PN
Short-term

The nurse responsible for the patient should be aware of the potential acute complications associated with PN and report promptly any abnormal signs to the clinician (Table 7.2). The nurse experienced in the therapy of PN can also guide the more inexperienced clinician, ensuring that routine blood tests and investigations are implemented on a regular basis. Some patients are at risk of particular complications, therefore all staff responsible for the PN patient should be vigilant for relevant signs and symptoms of mechanical and metabolic complications. For example, a large unexpected fluid loss from a fistula may require prompt adjustment to the electrolyte and fluid content of the PN. Sudden tachypnoea may be relevant to the administration of PN, due to fluid overload.

The need for frequent blood tests and venepuncture can be distressing

Table 7.2 Short-term metabolic complications associated with PN

Complication	Cause	Detection/treatment
Hyperosmolar coma Can occur acutely if a rapid infusion of hypertonic fluid is administered.	Infusion can cause severe osmotic diuresis, resulting in electrolyte abnormalities, dehydration and malfunction of the central nervous system.	Daily blood samples, accurate measurements of fluid balance, routine blood samples, reduce infusion rate, correct electrolyte imbalances.
Electrolyte imbalance Disturbances in serum electrolytes, particularly sodium, potassium, urea and creatinine, may occur early in the treatment of PN.	Often caused by patient's underlying medical condition; requirements vary depending on individual patient's needs. Can be caused by inadequate or excessive administration of intravenous fluids.	Daily blood samples taken early in treatment to detect abnormalities. Replacement fluid as required, extra intravenous fluids may be required during the stabilisation period.
Hyperglycaemia Disturbance of blood sugar.	Patients who are septic, traumatised or burned are resistant to insulin because of the secretion of ACTH and adrenaline. This promotes the secretion of glycogen, which inhibits the insulin response to hyperglycaemia (Frayn 1987).	Monitor patient's blood sugar 4-hourly after commencement of treatment, then daily when stable. Monitor daily urinalysis for glucose and ketones. Reduce the infusion rate of the feed bag. Sliding-scale insulin may be indicated until blood sugars stable.
Rebound hypoglycaemia On discontinuation of PN rebound hypoglycaemia may occur.	After prolonged intravenous nutrition hyperinsulinism occurs. A rise in serum insulin occurs with infusion and thus sudden cessation of infusion can result in hypoglycaemia.	Glucose infusion rate should be gradually reduced over the final hour of infusion before disconnecting infusion.
Hypophosphataemia Risk of developing hypophosphataemia. This may induce life-threatening complications.	Glucose infusion results in the continuous release of insulin, stimulating anabolism and resulting in rapid influx of phosphorus into muscle cells. The greatest risk is to malnourished patients with overzealous administration of feeding. Patients who are hyperglycaemic, who require insulin therapy during PN, or who have a history of alcoholism or chronic weight loss may require extra phosphate in the early stages of treatment.	Monitor phosphate levels daily. Usually appears after 24–48 h of treatment. Infusion rates of PN should be commenced slowly. If the patient does become hypophosphataemic, then the carbohydrate load should be decreased by reducing the PN. Phosphate supplementation should be given (Thompson & Hodges 1984).
Lipid clearance Can occur within 6 h of administration of lipid feed.	Lipids are broken down in the bloodstream with the aid of lipoprotein lipase found in the epithelium of capillaries in many tissues. A syndrome	Blood samples should be taken after the first infusion commences (within 6 h) to observe for lipid in the blood after commencement

Table 7.2 (contd)

Complication	Cause	Detection/treatment
	known as fat overload syndrome can occur when infusion of lipid is administered which is beyond the patient's clearing capacity, resulting in lipid deposits in the capillaries.	of treatment to ensure that lipid clearance has occurred.
Side-effects of lipid infusion Some patients suffer symptoms either during or after an infusion of lipid mix parenteral nutrition.	The exact cause is unknown. The patient may complain of headache, nausea or vomiting and generally feel unwell.	Inform patient of potential side-effects and treat mild symptoms. If tolerated the PN solution of non-protein calories can be given in the form of glucose. However, it is essential that the regime includes some fat to prevent the development of fatty acid deficiency.
Anaphylactic shock	This is a rare complication but may occur as a reaction to the administration of lipid.	In severe cases call the arrest team. It may be necessary to administer adrenaline/steroids.
Glucose intolerance Energy sources in PN may be in the form of glucose or fat. Using glucose as the prominent source of energy can result in respiratory distress.	PN using glucose as the main source of calories is associated with an increase in oxygen consumption and CO_2 production. The workload imposed by the high CO_2 production may precipitate respiratory distress in susceptible patients, particularly those requiring artificial ventilation.	Observe patients for signs of respiratory distress. Provide non-protein calories in the form of glucose lipid mix. Slow initial rate of infusion.
Liver function tests Abnormalities with liver function tests are associated with PN. They may level out or remain elevated for the duration of the treatment.	May be attributable to hepatic stenosis with moderate hepatomegaly, patient may also develop jaundice. Liver function tests often return to normal after cessation of therapy; however, PN can lead to severe hepatic dysfunction in neonates (Drongowski & Arnold 1989). Many clinicians believe that the development of abnormal liver functions are more likely the cause of the underlying medical problem.	Monitor liver function tests twice weekly. There are several factors which may contribute to development of abnormal liver function tests. These most often occur after a period of time and appear to be more of a problem when there is an excess calorie intake or in glucose-based PN regimens (Buchmiller et al 1993).

for the PN patient, particularly if venous access is a problem. Blood glucose monitoring may not only be painful for the patient requiring routine monitoring, but may also disrupt the patient's sleep pattern. Throughout this stage of treatment the nurse must be sensitive to the discomfort these investigations may cause to the patient. Reassurance that once stability is reached investigations reduce will often relieve the patient and his family.

Long-term

Patients requiring prolonged periods of PN may often experience complications specific to this type of nutrition.

Sepsis

Infection is undoubtedly the most serious complication associated with long-term PN. The avoidance and management of this will be discussed in great depth later in the chapter.

Gallstones

Prolonged use of PN can cause the formation of gallstones. Gallstones often appear to be more of a problem when the patient receives nothing via the enteral route, i.e. total PN as opposed to supplemental PN. Children would appear to have an increased incidence of gallstones.

Abdominal pain associated with a rise in serum bilirubin, whether in the presence or absence of jaundice, are indicators of possible gallstones. Gallstones may form in the biliary tract, where they cause an obstruction within the cystic duct. This results in pain, and thus the gallstones require removal.

Liver damage

An elevation of liver function tests is commonly seen at the commencement of PN. This is not liver damage as such, but is caused by the induction of enzymes for the metabolism of PN. Any abnormal liver function must be thoroughly investigated and the PN regimen reviewed with regard to lipid, carbohydrate and nitrogen content in order that further liver damage is avoided.

Trace element abnormalities

Metabolic complications associated with trace element deficiencies have been documented in patients receiving long-term PN. A routine screening protocol should be in place to detect such deficiencies and toxicity, with the PN solution adjusted accordingly to meet the patient's needs.

Metabolic bone disease

This may occur as a result of intestinal disease or steroid-related therapy. Patients on long-term PN should attend for bone density studies and treatment given if required.

OTHER NURSING ISSUES

The realisation of the inability to eat, however ill the patient may be, is often devastating for him and his family. This demoralising issue will require tact and diplomacy by the nurse in assuring the patient that, with nutritional support, this will often be a temporary state of affairs. Nurses will be instrumental in assisting and encouraging the patient requiring PN and they can be creative in ensuring that the patient's mobility, self-esteem and general confidence are developed.

Cyclical feeding

As the condition of the patient stabilises and the need for monitoring decreases the patient will enter a rehabilitation period. During this period of time the patient may benefit from cyclical feeding (overnight or a reduced period of time), which has physiological as well as psychological benefits, allowing the patient to become more mobile and improve his sense of wellbeing.

Advantages of cyclical feeding

Providing the patient with continuous PN is non-physiologic. The human body is not designed to receive nutrients continuously and has developed a system of storage where nutrients can be mobilised to be used when required once levels of insulin are reduced. With continuous feeding the body remains in a high insulin fed state, providing an opportunity to store nutrients instead of mobilising them. Excess glucose is converted to fat, which in turn can lead to fatty infiltration of the liver (Friel & Bistrian 1997). The use of cyclical feeding relieves the patient from the burden of constantly being attached to an intravenous infusion pump and stand. This method of administering PN has immense psychological benefits, encouraging a more normal daily pattern and a return to an independent lifestyle. It has been recognised that there is a link between the healing process and the patient's ability to participate in his own care.

Disadvantages of cyclical feeding

Cyclical feeding is not recommended in critically ill patients whose intolerance of glucose would not allow high rates of infusion. Patients experiencing unstable biochemistry and who therefore require frequent monitoring are another group who would be unsuitable for this type of administration. An increased infusional rate of PN can often increase the patient's urinary output, creating sleep disturbance – an important fact for any hospital patient.

Restricted enteral intake

Eating and drinking is an important part of human existence, providing social and psychological wellbeing. Meals are often pleasurable and social occasions. If the clinical condition of the patient prevents an enteral intake this can be a very difficult and distressing issue, causing physiological as well as psychological distress.

If the patient is required to remain nil by mouth it is important that the patient receives adequate hydration and appropriate measures are taken to relieve the dryness of the mouth. Provision of sips of water or small ice chips to suck if allowed will be received with great appreciation. Routine mouth care is vitally important for the patient unable to eat or drink; mouthwashes and oral hygiene should be provided as required. The patient's lips can become very dry and the application of vaseline or lip salve can be helpful. Giving the patient sweets to suck or small pieces of citrus fruit can encourage saliva production and the use of chewing gum, if tolerated, can also be helpful. It is very rare that the patient is unable to swallow even a small amount of water and the necessity for the patient to be completely nil by mouth needs to be reviewed regularly. Mealtimes can be particularly difficult and distressing for the patient when the smell of food is often a reminder of his clinical condition.

Patients receiving short-term PN recognise the period of nil by mouth will be short lived. However, the long-term PN patient may initially present a very resentful attitude to other patients' appreciation of food. Measures by the nursing staff encouraging the patient to avoid being present at mealtimes, possibly going for a shower or going to the dayroom to watch television, may help.

It is therefore very important for the nurse to be aware of these emotions, demonstrating sensitivity to the patient. It is also important for the nurse to make domestic and other ward staff aware that the patient should not receive oral diet, thus avoiding the patient being offered food inappropriately.

Reduction in mobility

The effect of the underlying illness and PN can affect the patient's motivation to mobilise. As the condition of the patient becomes more stable non-essential monitoring and general restrictions should be reduced.

It is very important that once the patient begins to mobilise he is actively encouraged to adopt a more normal routine. The use of portable drip stands allows the patient to be ambulant around the ward, and the use of portable infusion pumps gives an even greater flexibility. The use of cyclical feeding allows the patient to bath or shower, to dress and experience fewer restrictions on mobility. With prolonged treatment of PN the recovery period will involve the use of physiotherapy to improve the patient's strength and to assist in developing the patient's muscles. Creativity by the nursing staff will encourage the patient to experiment with his mobilisation and return to a normal lifestyle.

Change in body image

The patient receiving PN, particularly in the longer term, may have to cope with altered body image. Severe loss of weight, abnormal skin colouring, skin rashes and loss of hair are all examples of changes that may have occurred to the patient, particularly if he was malnourished prior to the commencement of PN. Each patient will perceive these changes differently and the care required to address body image will depend on the patient's individual needs. The central catheter itself may often add to the patient's perception of altered body image, particularly in those patients requiring long-term therapy.

Common symptoms include decreased socialisation, denial of changes, avoidance of physical contact with family and preoccupation with the change. The nurse will often act as confidante to the patient, and by encouraging the patient to discuss anxieties will often alleviate many preconceived ideas the patient may have. Suggestions can be made to improve physical appearance, for instance encouraging the patient to get dressed and adopt a regular, more normal routine. A visit by the hairdresser or the use of makeup can aid in raising the patient's morale following a period of hospitalisation. In some cases it may be helpful to involve a clinical psychologist or trained counsellor to assist the patient to work through anxieties associated with PN and provide methods to overcome them. National support groups (Patients on Intravenous and Nasogastric Nutrition Therapy, PINNT or 1/2 PINNT) may also provide the patient with an opportunity to meet other people experiencing similar difficulties whilst receiving PN.

Disturbance of sleeping pattern

The frequent monitoring and observation of the patient receiving PN can result in a disturbance of the patient's sleeping pattern. Over a period of time this can affect the patient both physically and mentally. In the early stages, when the patient is acutely unwell, or when treatment has just commenced, the disturbance is unavoidable. The nurse should be sensitive and flexible to the needs of the patient whenever practically possible. Encouraging the patient to sleep for short periods during the day may help, ensuring that during these periods the patient is not disturbed unnecessarily. Involving the patient with his own treatment and monitoring can be helpful, encouraging the patient to regain control of his life.

Transition to enteral feeding and oral diet

The transition from parenteral feeding to enteral feeding (EN) or oral diet is often advised using a dual approach, by reducing PN and increasing EN and oral intake gradually. Hospital food is invariably unappetising and a patient who has required PN over a period of time will be very unlikely to have any appetite.

This may cause anxiety and distress to the patient, particularly if he feels under pressure to eat. During this period there may also be other distressing symptoms. The patient may experience difficulty in ingesting food, suffer from diarrhoea, constipation, vomiting and a feeling of fullness. The last is a common complaint, particularly when the transition from PN to EN is taking place. This will often restrict the patient's willingness to eat as he will learn to associate food with upsetting symptoms. Cyclical feeding is often useful and less demoralising for the patient in this situation and will avoid the patient receiving PN and EN at the same time.

Reassurance by the nursing team and encouragement to eat small, frequent meals will reintroduce the patient to the pleasures of eating. Symptoms should be treated as they occur and gradually the patient's appetite will resume. Contact with a dietitian at this stage is particularly important with a diet plan arranged to meet the needs and desires of the patient. A food record chart will also aid the dietitian in assessing the patient's ability to tolerate an acceptable calorie intake and in determining the amount of enteral or parenteral feed that is required. A daily estimate of the patient's enteral intake will aid the NST in timing the withdrawal of PN and encouraging and maintaining EN.

GUIDELINES AND POLICIES FOR CATHETER MANAGEMENT

The most common complication associated with PN is infection. For this reason, great emphasis must be placed on the aseptic technique and management of the PN catheter, thus ensuring septic complications will be minimised. Staff caring for the patient receiving PN should have access to guidelines and policies to prevent complications occurring with the PN catheter. Guidelines should include the detection, prevention, and treatment of:

- infection

- central venous thrombosis
- catheter occlusion
- catheter damage.

Infection

Catheter-related sepsis is defined as:

'Clinical picture of spiking fever and chills resulting from blood passage of microorganisms from an intravascular infusion system. Isolation of the same organism from blood and catheter segments is considered definite proof' (Sitges-Serra et al 1995).

The teaching package for the inexperienced nurse or patient receiving HPN should include detailed discussion regarding the importance of infection control. The development of catheter-related sepsis is often via healthcare workers, either during preparation of PN, the dressing procedure, or during the administration process, and in particular when changing the PN. An understanding regarding the transmission of microorganisms is essential if the nurse or patient is to become competent in the care of the catheter. The skills of the nurse will be required to inform the patient of the safe management of PN and its potential complications, without increasing anxiety regarding therapy. Knowledge of the principles in the management and administration of PN is essential if errors are to be avoided.

There appears to be a common misconception that the environment provides the main risk for the transmission of microorganisms and that the patient is at greatest risk from the environment. This is in fact not the case, as microorganisms require a vector (the transport of a microbe) for their transmission, the most common of which is the skin and hands of staff and patients. Within the patient's vascular system microorganisms first need to establish a colonisation before an infection can occur. Microbes cannot multiply in a dry environment and most die rapidly. However, these microbes will multiply within the moist warm skin of individuals. This explains why transmission most frequently occurs by direct contamination from the skin of the patient, or that of the healthcare worker caring for the patient.

Pathophysiology of catheter-related sepsis

The protective barriers of the skin have been bypassed with the insertion of a catheter, providing a direct route for the entry of microorganisms into the vascular system. The catheter acts as a foreign body to the patient and can cause a local immune response. Within minutes of insertion a fibrin sheath may begin to form around the catheter (Hoshal et al 1971). This is formed from a collection of platelets and fibrin adhering to the tip of

---

Box 7.4 Mechanisms for the contamination of the catheter

- Introduced at catheter insertion.
- Migration of organisms down the external surface of the catheter via the exit site. Organisms usually originate from the patient's skin and flora.
- Catheter hub contamination during feed changes usually arises from organisms on staff. Higher risk with more manipulation of the catheter (Sitges-Serra et al 1984).
- Contaminated intravenous fluids occurring during the addition of vitamins to bag, allowing organisms to develop within the PN bag.
- Colonisation seeding from remote infection. Seeding may be caused by distant septic focus such as urinary tract infection. The importance has not been established and it is not thought to be a significant risk factor (Chuang & Chuang 1991).

---

the catheter. The fibrin sheath can be further complicated by a thrombus, which can provide a focus for the adherence of bacteria. Some bacteria such as *Staphylococcus epidermis* also produce an extracellular slime that enables them to adhere to and multiply on plastic and metal. The mechanisms for catheter contamination are listed in Box 7.4.

Main contaminants associated with PN catheters

Catheters used for PN can become contaminated by a variety of pathogens. The most common are *S. epidermis*, *Staphylococcus aureus*, Candida and enterococci (Larson 1995). The largest percentage of microorganisms isolated is *S. aureus* and *S. epidermis*, which suggests that the hands of health professionals and the flora of the patient's skin are the most likely sources of infection. There has also been the alarming emergence of vancomycin-resistant enterococci and methicillin-resistant *S. aureus*.

Detection and treatment of catheter-related sepsis (CRS)

The nurse should be vigilant for signs of CRS. These include the following (Second National Prevalence Survey of Infection in Hospitals 1993):

- *Exit site* – purulent discharge or exudation from the site of insertion, or a painful spreading erythema indicative of cellulitis.
- *Subcutaneous tunnel* – pain and/or spreading erythema over part or all of the area encompassing the subcutaneous catheter.
- *Systemic catheter-related sepsis* – fever >38°C, plus positive blood cultures. The results will be probable where no catheter tip culture is available, or definite where the blood culture and catheter tip yield indistinguishable bacterial isolates.

A protocol for the management of CRS should be available (Fig. 7.3). Despite clinical presentation of sepsis, it should not always be assumed

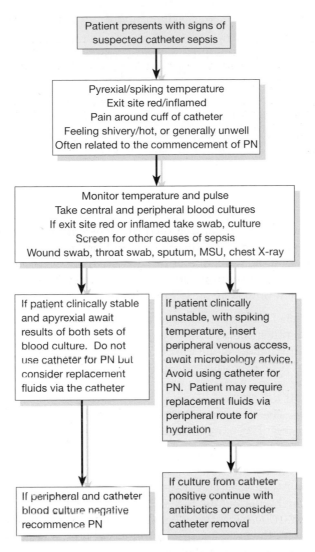

Fig. 7.3   Protocol for the management of catheter-related sepsis. MSU, midstream specimen of urine.

that the catheter is the cause. Other investigations should be carried out to prevent a catheter being removed unnecessarily. However, the catheter should not be used until the diagnosis of sepsis is confirmed. Whilst awaiting this the catheter should be flushed and heparinised to limit the formation of thrombus at the tip of the cvc, encouraging a focus for infection. The use of an infected catheter can have serious implications for the patient, as the microorganisms circulate in the vascular system and may even adhere to the valves of the heart, causing endocarditis. The decision on whether to use antibiotics to treat the sepsis or to remove the catheter immediately will be based on which type of microorganism is present, the continuing need for the catheter, available venous access, and future need for PN.

In the situation where CRS becomes an issue and there is limited available venous access in the patient requiring long-term PN, aggressive antibiotic therapy to preserve the existing venous access may be the only alternative.

Handwashing

The most common cause of the spread of nosocomial (hospital-acquired) infection is via the hands of healthcare workers due to poor handwashing standards. A discussion regarding the principles of handwashing and the appropriate use of gloves is therefore mandatory. Handwashing is the first crucial step in the reduction of catheter sepsis.

Microorganisms present on the skin can be categorised into transient flora and resident flora (Larson 1995).

- *Transient flora.* These are microorganisms that have been acquired via contact with other people or the environment and are easily contracted, particularly by hands, when the object touched is moist. The skin has antibacterial properties that prevent the transient microorganisms surviving for more than a few hours. However, during this time they can be passed to other people or objects.
- *Resident flora.* The skin supports the growth of a variety of microorganisms. These organisms survive deep in the skin within the hair follicles and are far more complex to eliminate.

The majority of transient flora can be removed by the mechanical practice of handwashing with soap and water. It is therefore essential that nursing staff wash their hands before and after patient contact. The use of soap and water is described as a social handwash. Resident flora, however, are not removed with the use of soap and water and therefore an antibacterial handwash is required. Removal of resident skin flora during routine care is not usually necessary as they are not readily transferred to other people or to surfaces, and most microorganisms may not be pathogenic. Procedures that are invasive, such as the use of intravenous catheters, are at risk from resident flora. This is frequently seen with the contamination of many catheters with *S. aureus*.

Any procedure connected with an intravenous catheter would require the nurse to wash with an antibacterial handwash, often described as antiseptic handwash. There are several types of antibacterial handwashes available for use (see Box 7.5), each having different properties and advantages. Choosing the appropriate agent will depend on several factors.

Box 7.5   Commonly used antiseptic handwashes

- Alcohol has good bacterial activity against most Gram-positive and Gram-negative microorganisms, tubercle bacillus, fungi and viruses. It provides the most rapid and greatest reduction in microbial count. Alcohol-based handwashes are not considered satisfactory cleaning agents and therefore are not recommended in the presence of physical dirt. Some alcohol concentrations can have a drying effect and can cause roughness of the skin.
- Chlorhexidine gluconate is more effective against Gram-negative bacteria, minimally against tubercle bacillus, fair against fungi, and active against a variety of viruses. It has a moderate speed in reductions of flora, but its main advantage is its persistence, as it can remain active for 6 h.
- Iodine/iodophors has a wide range of activity against Gram-negative and Gram-positive bacteria, tubercle bacillus, fungi and viruses. However, it can be neutralised in the presence of blood or sputum and can cause problems with skin irritations.

'APIC guideline for handwashing and hand antiseptics in healthcare settings' (Larson 1995) describes three stages:

- characteristics that are desired (e.g. rapid destruction in flora, spectrum of activity)
- evidence of safety and efficacy
- staff acceptance.

Practice of handwashing. The use of any form of antiseptic handwashes will prove to be ineffective if the correct handwashing technique is not employed. Various studies have concluded that healthcare workers do not wash their hands effectively, leaving many parts of the hands not exposed to soap and water or handwash. In practice the most commonly missed areas are the fingertips, the thumb and the inside of the fingers.

Details of the handwash should be clearly documented in the guidelines for recommended handwashing solution. When an antiseptic handwash has been performed the use of alcohol handrubs is effective. These can be applied quickly (15 to 20s) and will remove both transient and resident bacteria; however, it should be noted that handrubs should not be used if hands are visibly soiled.

Use of gloves. Gloves should not be used in place of handwashing. Many healthcare workers believe that gloves protect them and their patient from cross-contamination, but in reality this is not the case as hands can easily become contaminated under gloves if unwittingly punctured or when they are removed. It is recommended therefore that hands should be washed before and after the use of gloves. The use of sterile gloves for many procedures should be carefully examined. Nurses can give themselves a false sense of security with the use of gloves, which can easily become contaminated, and it may be more appropriate that the procedure is based on a non-touch technique, thus eliminating the need for sterile gloves.

Nursing care of the PN catheter

Monitoring the exit site of the cvc. Following insertion of any cvc, careful monitoring of both incision and exit sites is required. There may be leakage of blood around the exit site requiring regular changes of dressing after the first 24 h to ensure the exit site of the catheter remains free of serum and blood. If left, this will create a focus for infection that potentially can track back, entering the subcutaneous tunnel, and in this way gaining access to the vascular system.

Dressing the feeding catheter. Following cvc insertion it is often advisable in the first 24 h to add to the original dressing, encouraging clot formation. Aseptic replacement of the original dressing may then be performed the following day.

The key to the prevention of exit site infection appears to be the cleansing technique and the choice of dressing. It is generally recommended that antiseptics are used to clean the site. Maki et al (1991) suggest in their study of skin cleansing agents that chlorhexidine 2% is the most effective, providing the solution is allowed to dry. The use of acetone to defat the skin, which has the effect of removing microorganisms from lipids on the skin surface, was also studied by Maki & McCormack (1987). However, this has not been proven worthwhile. The use of topical antibiotics, although reducing the rate of sepsis, is not recommended owing to the associated high risk of fungal infection. A suggested method for dressing the feeding catheter is outlined in Box 7.6.

Most studies recommend changing dressings at 48 h intervals, or if the catheter exit is no longer airtight. Assessment of the exit site at dressing changes is particularly important to detect any sign of redness, inflammation or exudate. Any changes noted should be documented and communicated to other colleagues and the nurse within the NST.

Common dressings used are sterile gauze, adhesive gauze or transparent occlusive dressing. There has been some concern about the use of the latter due to the moisture build-up within the dressing and the potential for

---

Box 7.6 Method for dressing the feeding catheter

- Using a non-touch, aseptic technique, the exit site of the feeding catheter should be cleansed with an alcoholic based solution.
- Using a circular movement, starting from the centre and working away from the catheter will ensure that any skin organisms are encouraged away from the exit site. During the cleansing process, movement of the catheter should be limited to prevent unnecessary trauma.
- The cleaning procedure should be repeated, finally allowing the solution to dry. The cleansing solution must be allowed to dry naturally, enabling the action of the solution to achieve maximum potential prior to the application of the dressing.
- Once dry, the dressing may be applied to the exit site, ensuring the catheter is airtight and secure.

an increase in microorganism colonisation. Some studies have shown an increased rate of infection, while others have found no significant increase in sepsis rate. More recently a dressing has been developed that reduces the accumulation of moisture under the dressing, and a study by Kennlyside (1993) suggested that this dressing performed favourably when compared with an alternative transparent dressing. The use of dressings at all is questioned by some staff. In one study where no application of a dressing occurred after the catheter had been in place for 3 weeks, less infection was recorded in catheters with no dressing (Lucas & Attard-Montalto 1996). In another study there was no statistical difference when four types of dressing groups were studied; indeed, the group with no dressing performed slightly better (Petrisino et al 1988). It appears that the sepsis rate is far more likely to be affected by the experience and skills of the staff carrying out the procedures (Nelson et al 1986) than by the dressing used.

If a dressing is to be used, then the frequency of dressing a PN catheter will be determined by local protocol. Where a dressing is used to cover the exit site of the cvc, it should be airtight and free of exudate.

As studies have not been conclusive, it is for the nurse to make a clinical decision on which to base her guidelines or procedures. This should be based on the principles of the ideal dressing (Box 7.7).

Sutures. The incision made at the cannulation point, often below the clavicle, is usually sutured. The sutures will require removal after 5–7 days. If paper steristrips are used these can also be removed after a similar period of time. During this period ensuring both the cannulation site and the exit sites remain dry will aid the healing process, reduce the risk of infection and ensure limited scarring.

The suture that restricts movement of the catheter at the exit point will vary depending on the type of catheter inserted. If short-term PN is indicated, it is often considered more appropriate to insert a 'non-cuffed' feeding catheter. Only on cessation of PN will the restraining suture at the exit site be cut and the catheter removed. However, for prolonged use

---

Box 7.7   Properties of the ideal dressing for a PN catheter

- Sterile
- Prevents trauma to the catheter site
- Prevents contamination of the site
- Allows the exit site to be visible
- Secures the catheter
- Comfortable for the patient
- Cost-effective
- Reduced frequency of change
- Keeps wound dry
- Easy to apply and remove

of PN a 'cuffed' feeding catheter may be considered to be a safer option. In this case the Dacron cuff of the catheter will fibrose within the subcutaneous tunnel, creating a mesh of fibres, ensuring secure venous access. The process of fibrosis may take up to 3 weeks to occur, during which time a suture around the catheter at the exit site will ensure the catheter does not become displaced. This is particularly important in patients requiring steroids, where the fibrosing action may be delayed. It is important that there is documentation of the type of catheter inserted, sutures used, and when they should be removed. A protocol determining these issues is often helpful.

Care of the catheter hub. Several studies have implicated contamination of the hub as the major source of catheter-related sepsis in catheters that remain in situ for more than 2 weeks. Sitges-Serra et al (1984) was concerned about the hub and recommended that limited manipulations to the catheter should occur, as each junctional break brings additional risk of infection. The single-lumen catheter should be used solely for the administration of PN and should not be used for the administration of drug therapy, additional intravenous fluids or for routine blood samples. If a multilumen catheter is used, one lumen (usually the distal) should be designated solely for PN. The remaining lumens should also receive similar scrupulous care and attention. Meticulous care must be taken when a break in the closed system occurs, including changing of the infusion set or when the catheter is flushed.

Clearly written, research-based guidelines pertinent to the clinical area will provide a useful resource for nurses managing the care of patients receiving PN via a cvc. This is of particular importance in departments of haematology, where chemotherapy and high-dose antibiotics are administered in close proximity to PN, creating even greater potential for catheter contamination.

Some centres have recommended the use of closed Luer lock connection devices with membranes to permit access to the catheter whilst maintaining a 'closed system' (bioconnector™, Interlink™, click lock™). However, such systems can be expensive, and with respectful nursing care of the catheter infection can be minimised without the costs incurred from such devices.

The perceived benefit of the closed system is the prevention of catheter-related sepsis, reduction in use of sterile equipment, reduction in needle stick injuries and reduction in nursing workload and costs. There are very few studies available that report a significant reduction in CRS, although Segura et al (1996) did demonstrate a reduction in the rate of sepsis when a new catheter hub was introduced. In a local study we introduced new protocols using (Interlink™) which proved to be cost-effective and reduced nursing workload, with no increase in catheter-related sepsis (McWhirter et al 1997). Anecdotal evidence suggests that using the closed system is much less cumbersome for nursing staff and patients to use and compliance with the procedures may be better. The use of the closed systems does not diminish the need for careful catheter techniques; the adherence of staff to guidelines appears to be a vital aspect in the rate of sepsis.

The delivery system

A pharmacist should be responsible for supervision of the preparation of PN bags. Any additions to the bag should occur in a suitable compounding department with experienced pharmacy technicians. The pharmacy department adheres to aseptic dispensing guidelines documented in the Farwell report (1995). The aim of this report is to ensure that the facilities used are maintained to a high standard, there is close monitoring of the service provided, and an ongoing training programme for staff involved in providing the service is available.

The PN bags will usually require to be stored in the refrigerator until use. Incorrect storage may result in PN at incorrect temperature and contamination may occur. Before commencing PN the nurse should check the expiry date. The bag should also be checked for leaks, cracks, particulate matter or deposits. If present, the bag should not be used and the pharmacy department contacted for advice and possible replacement.

Contamination of the PN bag with particulate matter has been recorded and can have serious repercussions. This can come from debris, from reconstructed drugs or from additives in the solution. The presence of particles can place the patient at severe risk of contamination, which can cause a local reaction of phlebitis (Colagiavanni 1997). It was with this in mind that in-line filters were first introduced to prevent such debris entering the vascular system. However, the use of filters is now controversial and opinion is divided on their cost-effectiveness.

The main risk within the delivery system occurs during manipulation. The use of a closed administration system with reduced manipulation can reduce the risk of contamination with the intravenous system. Intravenous sets should only be changed after the discontinuation of PN or within certain limits (Box 7.8).

Box 7.8   Recommendations for changing administration sets

- Ideally use new administration set daily
- Can be used for 48 h if the system remains intact
- Change administration set immediately following blood transfusion
- Never administer blood via a PN catheter

Messner & Gorse (1987) recommend the following measures to reduce extrinsic contamination during the administration of PN:

- Preparation and mixing of PN solutions should be performed using aseptic technique and laminar airflow conditions.
- Manipulations of the closed administration system, including additions of vitamins, etc. to the PN bag, should be minimised.
- Administration sets should be changed at least every 48 h, preferably daily.
- The aspiration of blood via the PN catheter should be avoided. This practice encourages both infection and thrombus formation.
- Aseptic technique must be used when handling catheter junctions, with the handler wearing sterile gloves.
- Close inspection of all the administration equipment for hairline cracks or damage should be carried out.

Detection, prevention and treatment of venous thrombosis

Central venous thrombosis (CVT) is a serious complication of PN. It was initially thought to be an uncommon problem. However, many clinicians now believe that the occurrence is far more common than was first realised. Pithie et al (1988) reported an incidence of 16.8%. The use of prolonged PN and the introduction of HPN has seen an increase in the problem, which can have potentially serious repercussions.

Predisposing factors to CVT

The following factors predispose to CVT:

- The development of fibrin sleeves. Indwelling vascular catheters can develop a totally circumferential fibrin sleeve within 24 h of insertion (Hoshal et al 1971). Fibrin deposition can occur at the catheter insertion site extending over a period of days, eventually encapsulating the tip of the catheter. Fibrin can also form at the catheter tip and extend up the catheter towards the cannulation site. Within 5–7 days the entire length of the catheter can become encased in fibrin, and may contribute to the development of thrombus production.
- Vascular endothelial damage. The presence of an indwelling catheter can cause damage to the vein wall due to the tip of the catheter being positioned close to the intima of the vein.
- Infusion fluid. The administration of hyperosmolar solution of PN, particularly into the innominate vein, which is smaller than the subclavian or cephalic veins, can also predispose to thrombosis (Fabri et al 1982).

- Catheter type. The type of catheter material will often influence the occurrence of CVT. Thrombosis appears to be more common in polyvinyl catheters than in silicone catheters, as silicone catheters appear less thrombogenic. It is essential that the correct gauge of catheter is selected relative to the size of the vein, thus encouraging a brisk circulation of blood around the catheter.

Signs and symptoms of CVT

Early signs of venous thrombosis may be a less efficient performance from the catheter plus an erratic flow if aspiration is attempted. Clinical signs of venous thrombosis include engorgement of the upper limbs and neck veins, together with collateral venous distribution on the chest wall, which may be unilateral. There may be cyanosis, breathlessness and oedema. In the more extreme event of superior vena cava (svc) thrombosis, a mottled appearance of the neck and ears can also be noted. The diagnosis is confirmed with a venography and may require intravascular antifibrinolytic therapy.

Prevention and treatment

The use of heparin within the PN bag has been suggested at 1 iu/ml. However, this has not been shown to be effective (Bozzetti et al 1983) and may create instability of the nutrients. Although larger doses may be effective, the clinician has to take into account the potential side-effects larger doses of heparin may have on the patient, such as osteoporosis and the risk of bleeding. However, in those patients requiring long-term PN, low-dose anticoagulant therapy may be indicated.

Regular installation of urokinase via the catheter often aids in maintaining catheter patency in the long-term PN patient. Other preventative measures include the use of the least thrombogenic catheters such as silicone or polyurethane plus using catheters with the smallest lumen placed in the largest vein possible. When venous occlusion occurs the patient may be treated, depending on the severity of the occlusion, with heparin or thrombolytic agents such as streptokinase or tPA (tissue plasminogen activator) (Pennington 1991).

Catheter occlusion

Causes

Occlusion can occur within the lumen of the vein. This can be caused by any of the following:

- fibrin deposits caused by the formation of a clot due to stagnate blood which has been left within the lumen of the catheter;

- lipid sludge caused by the formation of lipid deposits;
- collection of amorphous debris;
- mechanical occlusion if the catheter is malpositioned, or a kink in the catheter has occurred;
- the formation of a fibrin sheath at the tip of the catheter can act as a one-way valve, allowing saline to be flushed but preventing the withdrawal of blood into the catheter (Gabriel 1997).

Factors to consider when attempting to avoid the incidence of intraluminal occlusion

There are several factors to consider when attempting to avoid intraluminal occlusion:

- catheter material
- occlusion due to static blood or nutrient solution
- catheter size
- protocol for flushing the catheter
- catheter design.

The material from which the catheter is made affects the propensity for the development of a thrombus within the catheter. It is unclear as to why some catheter materials are more thrombogenic than others, although it would appear that an uneven surface attracts platelet and bacterial adhesion, producing a turbulent and erratic blood flow that encourages thrombosis.

It is essential to prevent static blood or nutrient solution from occluding the lumen of the catheter. Various methods to avoid this occurrence have been employed such as the addition of heparin to the PN, heparin-coated catheters and most importantly, sodium chloride flush followed by heparin flush and lock after discontinuation of therapy.

To help prevent the occurrence of thrombosis, it is essential that an appropriate gauge catheter is selected relative to the size of the patient's vein. Ideally, a fine-bore catheter situated in the largest vein possible will encourage a high circulating blood volume, thus reducing the risk of thrombus formation at the tip of the catheter.

The use of antithrombotic agents in the maintenance of PN catheter patency is conflicting and opinions divided. Nicholl (1990) discusses personal experiences regarding the most effective methods of maintaining catheter patency. When the patient is receiving cyclical feeding, e.g. overnight feeding, heparinising the catheter after the discontinuation of therapy has been widely used as a preventative measure.

Some studies have recommended the use of saline as opposed to heparin (Epperson 1984, Garrelts et al 1989). The use of sodium chloride reduces costs and eliminates the potential anticoagulation side-effects of heparin.

Both these studies suggest that saline is as effective as heparin at maintaining patency of the catheter; however, neither study measured the bacterial colonisation of the catheter, which is thought to be reduced with the use of heparin.

When designing protocols for flushing central venous PN catheters, the interaction of heparin and calcium should be recalled. Rattenbury et al (1989) have suggested that heparin–calcium interactions due to paediatric all-in-one mixes were one of the major causes of catheter occlusion. The NST pharmacist may assist in the design of such a protocol and will advise on the most appropriate flushing routine for PN catheters.

The practice of flushing lines varies widely within the UK. A survey by Cottee (1995) was carried out to determine the current practice used to maintain catheter patency within the UK. The majority used heparin solution, although concentrations varied from 1 iu/ml to 5000 iu/ml, and the volumes used varied from 1 ml to 5 ml. Guidelines to maintain patency of PN catheters should be available, although current research is not available to determine the exact type and amount of fluid required to maintain patency. A low dose of heparin should be used to prevent associated complications.

The design of the catheter is also important in reducing the risk of thrombosis. PN catheters are now available that have a one-way valve, preventing the back-flow of blood into the catheter The manufacturers suggest that, owing to the presence of the valve, a heparin lock is no longer necessary when this type of catheter is used.

Nursing care required to reduce incidence of catheter occlusion

Whether nurse or patient become responsible for the management of the PN catheter, great importance must be placed on the reliability and patency of the catheter. Following insertion, the catheter should be flushed with heparinised saline, thus minimising the risk of prompt platelet formation at the tip of the catheter.

Once the cvc is inserted it is important that the catheter is flushed by the operator, leaving a heparinised 'lock' in place to reduce the formation of thrombus. Similarly, immediately after the completion of PN the catheter should be flushed first with sodium chloride, followed by heparinised saline.

In many cases occlusion is not sudden and is recognised by an increasing pressure required to flush the catheter. The nurse or patient must be made aware of the importance of regular flushing of the PN catheter to avoid the risk of catheter occlusion. Regular and systematic flushing of the PN catheter will aid in the prevention of catheter occlusion and possible loss of the catheter due to fibrin formation (see Fig. 7.4).

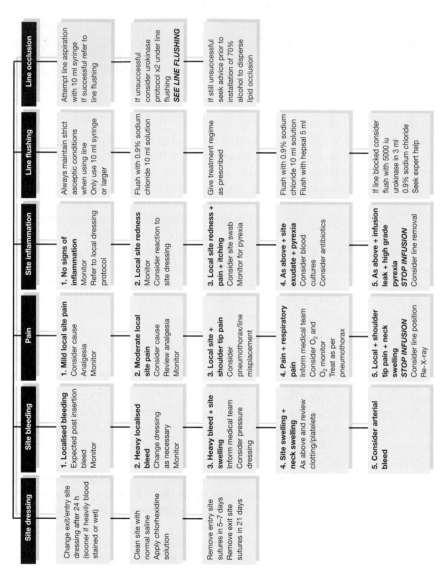

Fig. 7.4 Guidelines for management of catheters used for PN. (Provided by Steve McManus.)

Detection of occlusion

In the past the most common treatment available for an occluded catheter was to remove the catheter. However, with experience many catheters can be salvaged if preventative measures are taken.

When diagnosing an occluded catheter, it is important to determine whether there is a mechanical cause, for example a kink in the tubing, or a section of the catheter that is in an inappropriate position. The administration set should be removed from the pump to ensure that the pump is not malfunctioning. Using a process of elimination to determine the reason for the catheter occlusion can usually be productive.

If the catheter remains blocked, the following technique is suggested:

- Using an aseptic technique the catheter should gently be aspirated.
- This can be followed by gently flushing the catheter with sodium chloride.

Forceful flushing may rupture the catheter and cause very serious problems for the patient, e.g. transitory air embolus, loose foreign body entering the vascular circulation, extravasation, etc. No force must ever be exerted in this manner and any temptation to do this must be resisted.

- Syringes smaller than 10 ml should never be used owing to the increased pressure that can be exerted on the catheter.
- Gentle flushing with sodium chloride may be enough to unblock a catheter.

However, for the more stubborn occlusions a chest X-ray may be useful in determining whether any kinks in the catheter are present. The tip of the catheter may be lodged against the vein wall. While enabling flushing, this will not yield blood. If the catheter remains occluded and the type of occlusion is diagnosed, a suitable agent is often required to dissolve the occlusion.

Treatment of occlusion

Clearly, it is important at this stage to establish what has caused the occlusion. Central venous catheters may obstruct not only as a result of thrombus, but also due to the accumulation of lipid or chemical debris within the catheter lumen.

Fibrin deposits. Fibrin occlusion may respond to the administration of urokinase. This is an enzyme that functions by converting plasminogen to plasmin, which degrades fibrin and fibrinogen as well as other plasma proteins. Plasminogen is contained within and is also found on the surface of thrombus and emboli. Therefore, urokinase should act effectively in resolving a fibrin occlusion.

Installation of 5000 iu urokinase/3 ml sodium chloride into the affected catheter lumen, left for a minimum of 3 h, often aids in the dispersion of a fibrin occlusion. However, this therapy should be adopted with caution in those conditions associated with a high risk of bleeding or active bleeding.

Lipid deposits. The use of lipid 3 in 1 mixes has caused the presence of lipid deposits within the lumen of the catheter. The catheter can often perform sluggishly over a period of 2–3 days before becoming completely blocked. This behaviour is often indicative of lipid occlusion.

Pennington & Pithie (1987) have found that catheter occlusions due to lipid accumulation have responded well to 70% ethanol, instilled for 1 h prior to flushing. The use of 70% ethanol solution, which causes the lipid material to dissolve, can often aid in clearing the catheter of lipid deposits (Pennington 1991).

Locally we have replaced a saline flush with a 20% ethanol flush following lipid infusions, which in the majority of cases has prevented the problem of lipid occlusion (Tait et al 1997). Some centres infuse the lipid infusion separately in an attempt to prevent this problem. However, this is time-consuming and the practicalities of this system for the patient receiving HPN are more difficult.

Catheter damage

Catheter damage is more of a problem with long-term catheters, when the frequent clamping and unclamping of the catheter can result in rupture. However, there is the potential for it to occur at any time for a variety of reasons. One of the dangers associated with catheter damage is the risk of air and microorganisms gaining entry into the patient's vascular system. For this reason early recognition is of paramount importance.

Another concern, particularly for the patient receiving long-term PN, is the traumatic severing of the cvc, whereupon, bleeding can present a serious risk of haemorrhage. Careful observation of the catheter for leakage, particularly when the infusion commences or when the catheter is flushed after discontinuation of PN, is important, with prompt action necessary by the nursing team.

In the event of catheter fracture a non-traumatic clamp should be applied over gauze, preventing further damage to the catheter. The catheter may be repaired by experienced staff using a repair kit. However, this measure is often temporary. A repaired catheter can often function successfully for many months, but the risk of infection from the repaired site is always a concern and eventually the catheter will need to be replaced.

REFERENCES

Anderson DC, Heimburger DC, Morgan SL et al 1996 Metabolic complications of total parenteral nutrition: effects of a Nutrition Support Service. Journal of Parenteral and Enteral Nutrition 20 (3):201–210

Bozzetti F, Scarpa D, Terno G et al 1983 Subclavian venous thrombosis due to indwelling catheters: a prospective study on 52 patients. Journal of Parenteral and Enteral Nutrition 7:560–563

Buchmiller CE, Kleiman-Wexler RL, Ephgrave KS, Booth B, Hensley CE 1993 Liver dysfunction and energy source: Results of a randomised clinical trial. Journal of Parenteral and Enteral Nutrition 17 (4): 301–306

Burns D 1992 Working up a thirst … hospitalised patients' basic daily minimum fluid requirements. Nursing Times 88 (26):44–45

Chuang JH, Chuang SF (1991) Implication of a distant septic focus in parenteral nutrition catheter colonisation. Journal of Parenteral and Enteral Nutrition 15(2):173–175

Colagiavanni L 1997 Parenteral nutrition and in line filtration. Nursing Times 93 34 supplement

Cottee S 1995 Heparin lock practice in total parenteral nutrition. Professional Nurse 11(1):25–29

Daffurn K, Hillman KM, Bauman A, Lum M, Crispin C, Ince L 1994 Fluid balance charts: do they measure up? British Journal of Nursing 3(16):816–820

Drongowski RA, Arnold GC 1989 An analysis of factors contributing to the development of total parenteral nutrition induced cholestasis. Journal of Parenteral and Enteral Nutrition 13:586–589

Epperson EL 1984 Efficacy of 0.9% sodium chloride injection with and without heparin for maintaining indwelling intermittent injection sites. Clinical Pharmacy 3:626–629

Fabri PJ, Mirtallo JM, Ruberg RL et al 1982 Incidence and prevention of thrombosis of the subclavian vein during total parenteral nutrition. Surgery Gynecology and Obstetrics 155:238–240

Farwell J 1995 Aseptic dispensing for NHS patients. HMSO, London

Frayn KN 1987 Fuel metabolism during sepsis and injury. Intensive Therapy and Clinical Monitoring Nov/Dec 174–180

Friel C, Bistrian B 1997 Cycled total parenteral nutrition; is it more effective? American Journal of Clinical Nutrition 65:1078–1079

Gabriel J 1997 Fibrin sheaths in vascular access devices. Nursing Times 93 (10):56–57

Garrelts JC, La Rocca J, Ast D, Smith DF, Sweet DE 1989 Comparison of heparin and 0.9% sodium chloride injection in the maintenance of indwelling intermittent IV devices. Clinical Pharmacy 8 (1):34 39

Hoshal VL, Ause RG, Hoskins PA, Mich A 1971 Fibrin sleeve formation in indwelling subclavian central venous catheters. Archives of Surgery 102:353–358

Kennlyside D 1993 Avoiding an unnecessary outcome. Professional Nurse Feb 288–291

Larson EL 1995 APIC guideline for handwashing and hand antiseptics in health care settings. American Journal of Infection Control 23(4):251–269

Lucas H, Attard-Montalto S 1996 The effectiveness of dressings in reducing exit site infection following central venous catheterisation. Paediatric Nursing 8 (6):21–23

McWhirter JP, Tait J, Pennington CR 1997 Interlink reduces the cost of cylical parenteral nutrition. Proceedings Nutrition Society 56(2):246A

Maki DG, McCormack KN 1987 Defatting catheter insertion sites in Total Parenteral Nutrition is of no value as an infection control measure. American Journal of Medicine 83(5):833–840

Maki DG, Ringer M, Alvarado CJ 1991 Prospective randomised trial of providone-iodine, alcohol and chlorhexidine for prevention of infection associated with central venous and arterial catheters. Lancet 338:339–342

Meers P, Jacobsen W, McPherson M 1992 Hospital infection control for nurses. Chapman & Hall, London, p 36

Messuer RL, Gorse GJ 1987 Nursing management of peripheral intravenous sites. Focus on Critical Care 14(2): 25–33

Methany NM 1996 Fluid and electrolyte balance nursing considerations. Lippincott, New York, p 32

Mughal MM 1989 Complications of intravenous feeding catheters. British Journal of Surgery 76:15–21

Nelson DB, Kien CL, Mohr B, Frank S, Davis SD 1986 Dressing changes by specialised personnel reduce the infection rates in patients receiving central venous parenteral nutrition. Journal of Parenteral and Enteral Nutrition 10(2):220–222

Nicholl LH 1990 Heparin vs saline debate. American Journal of Nursing 90(9): 27

Pennington CR 1991 Parenteral nutrition: the management of complications. Clinical Nutrition 10:133–137

Pennington CR, Pithie AD 1987 Ethanol lock in the management of catheter occlusion. Journal of Parenteral and Enteral Nutrition 11(5):507–508

Petrisino B, Becker H, Christian B 1988 Infection rates in central venous catheter dressings. Oncology Nursing Forum 15(6):709–717

Pithie A, Soutar JS, Pennington CR (1988) Catheter tip position in central venous thrombosis. Journal of Parenteral and Enteral Nutrition 12(6):613–614

Rattenbury JM, Timmins JG, Cawthorne EA, Ganapathy S, Taylor CJ 1989 Identification of the cause of separation (creaming) of lipid emulsions in intravenous infusion. Journal of Paediatric Gastroenterology and Nutrition 8(4): 491–495

Second National Prevalence Survey of Infection in Hospitals 1993 Co-ordinating Centre University Hospital, Nottingham

Segura M, Alvarez-Lerma F, Tellado JM, et al 1996 A clinical trial of the prevention of catheter related sepsis using a new hub model. Annals of Surgery 223 (4):363–369

Sitges-Serra A, Linares J, Garau J 1984 Catheter sepsis: the clue is the hub. Surgery 97(3):355–357

Sitges-Serra A, Pi-Serra T, Garces JM, Segura M 1995 Pathogenesis and prevention of catheter related septicemia. American Journal of Infection Control 23 (5):310–316

Tait JM, Baxter JP, Pennington CR 1998 Review of protocols to prevent catheter occlusion. Proceedings of the Nutrition Society 57:107A

Thompson JS, Hodges RE 1984 Preventing hypophosphataemia during total parenteral nutrition. Journal of Parenteral and Enteral Nutrition 82:137–139

United Kingdom Central Council for Nursing Midwifery and Health Visiting (UKCC) 1992a The Code of Professional Practice. UKCC, London

United Kingdom Central Council for Nursing Midwifery and Health Visiting (UKCC) 1992b The Scope of Professional Practice. UKCC, London

8

Dietetic aspects of parenteral nutrition

Helen Dewar

Introduction
Assessing the appropriateness of referral
Considerations when starting PN
Dietetic monitoring

Nutritional complications of PN
Weaning from PN
Conclusion

INTRODUCTION

As described in Chapter 1, enteral nutrition (EN) is where nutrition is provided directly to the gastrointestinal (GI) tract whether it is taken orally or via a tube. Parenteral nutrition (PN) is when a patient is fed directly into the circulatory system via a central venous catheter or peripheral vein. When a patient is referred for PN it is important that a detailed assessment is made. The importance and desirability of EN cannot be overemphasised.

EN performs more than one task: not only does it provide sufficient nutrients for the body, but it also preserves the structure of the gut. When disused, the cells lining the GI tract slough away and leave a 'leaky gut'. Bacterial translocation can then occur, that is the movement of bacteria from the gut to other systems, e.g. lymph. This has been proved in animal models, but is still controversial in humans. However, it is likely that the toxins produced by the bacteria can translocate as they are smaller and more able to move between the gaps in the gut cells. Bacterial and/or toxin translocation is thought to play an important role in the development of multiple organ failure.

Another advantage of EN is a reduction in nosocomial infection. With lack of enteral stimulation the gall bladder becomes stagnant, causing sludging that can lead to stone formation. The liver is also adversely affected; liver function tests will be mentioned in more detail later in the chapter. For these reasons, if it is possible, a small amount of EN should be encouraged, e.g. on the intensive care unit (ICU) 10 ml/h of feed is thought to be sufficient to keep the gut cells stimulated and help prevent gall bladder stasis.

ASSESSING THE APPROPRIATENESS OF REFERRAL

Due to the risks associated with PN, including central line placement, PN is not normally considered to be of benefit unless it is required for more than 7–10 days. For shorter periods of time the risk of inserting a central line outweighs the benefit gained by short-term PN.

Therefore PN should only be considered when:

- All routes of EN have been investigated and dismissed as clinically inappropriate (this has been covered in detail in Ch. 3).
- Total gut rest is needed, e.g. acute pancreatitis, small bowel fistulae, gastrochiasis, exomphalos.
- If the GI tract is inaccessible, e.g. oesophageal fistula or stricture, when it is not possible to insert an enteral feeding tube.
- Total nutritional requirements cannot be met enterally owing to a decreased ability to absorb nutrients, e.g. short bowel syndrome.
- EN will not be possible for a period of at least 7–10 days or more.
- The patient's prognosis is good, and she will only transiently require PN, or will be able to sustain a good quality of life on PN, if it is necessary long term, e.g. short bowel syndrome.

Both short-term and long-term goals for PN should be identified to ensure that PN is used for the right reasons and not prolonged beyond this goal out of convenience.

The key message is that PN should not be entered into lightly. Although it can be a life-saving therapy, it is expensive and has potentially life-threatening complications. Therefore where possible the enteral route should be used. Parenteral nutritional support is indicated if EN is not possible or not clinically indicated, the situation is unlikely to be resolved within a week, and the patient is initially malnourished. As discussed in Chapter 7, when PN is commenced it is important that it is administered correctly and closely monitored. EN should be introduced as soon as clinically possible so as not to subject the patient to invasive feeding for longer than necessary.

CONSIDERATIONS WHEN STARTING PN

PN should not be considered as an emergency procedure in adults, and patients should be carefully prepared before a central venous catheter (cvc) is inserted (Ch. 5). The use of short-term peripheral feeds, such as Vitrimix or Clinimix, can be used for short-term administration of PN. This is particularly useful over a weekend period. However, these solutions lack vitamins, minerals and trace elements, and the electrolytes and volume are not tailored for individual patient requirements.

Dietetic assessment

Once a patient has been accepted for PN there are a number of factors to consider before setting up the PN bag. Past medical history and current presenting complaint may indicate that the patient has additional problems needing a more specialised bag of PN. For example:

- Patients experiencing liver/renal failure may require specific tailoring of nutrients including protein/nitrogen, fluid and electrolytes. This group of patient may also require certain types of lipid to avoid further complications associated with metabolism.
- Those experiencing large stoma losses, or fluid and electrolyte imbalances, require correction before PN is commenced. However, if PN is in progress extra fluid can be administered via a side-arm administration set, aseptically plumbed in the pharmacy department with a Y-connector to the PN system.

Details of the electrolyte content of intravenous fluids and the approximate electrolyte solutions of various body fluids are given in Tables 8.1 and 8.2.

The dietitian will assess the calorie and nitrogen requirement of the patient, based on age, gender, current weight, clinical condition and activity level (Todorovick & Micklewright 1997). The assessment is then discussed with the other members of the Nutrition Support Team (NST) in conjunction with the medical team. Most patients can normally receive a 'standard bag' of PN. This bag will vary from hospital to hospital, but will generally provide 2000–2400 kcal (1 kcal – 4.184 kJ) and 12–14 g nitrogen (75–88 g protein, where 1 g N is equivalent to 6.25 g protein) in 2 or 2.5 litres of fluid.

Hospitals with their own pharmacy aseptic service unit (ASU) may manufacture their own PN bags. However, even in these cases the pharmacy will encourage the use of a range of standard bags where possible.

Table 8.1 Electrolyte content of intravenous replacement fluids

	Sodium (mmol/L)	Potassium (mmol/L)	Chloride (mmol/L)
Normal saline	150	0	150
Dextrose saline (4% dextrose, 0.18% saline)	30	0	30
Hartmann's solution	131	5	131

Table 8.2 Approximate electrolyte solutions of various bodily fluids

	Gastric juice	Pancreatic juice	Bile	Ileostomy	Colostomy	Diarrhoea
Sodium (mmol/L)	15	130	145	50	60	30–140
Potassium (mmol/L)	140	5	5	4	15	30–70
Chloride (mmol/L)	0–15	55	100	25	40	–
Bicarbonate (mmol/L)	2–3	110	38	–	–	20–80
Volume (L/24 h)		0.5–1.0	0.5–1.0	0.5	0.1–0.2	

(After Lee 1974, with permission.)

Table 8.3 Body mass index (BMI) interpretation

BMI	Interpretation
<20	Undernourished
20–24.9	Adequately nourished
25–29.9	Overweight
>30	Obese

(After Garrow 1981, with permission.)

Standard bags are considerably more economical than individualised bags, which involve more pharmaceutical time and therefore more on-costs to the PN preparation. Hospitals without their own ASU will buy in PN bags from commercial companies. These companies usually also supply and deliver PN for patients on home PN.

It is important to establish the patient's weight and weight history and to assess if she is malnourished. Body mass index (BMI) is measured as weight in kilograms divided by the square of the height in metres. BMI is interpreted in various ranges, as shown in Table 8.3. This is a useful way of expressing a patient's height and weight and determining her nutritional state. This index reflects if weight loss or gain is needed. If a patient has a BMI of over 30, then the weight for calculation is taken at 75% of actual weight because the excess weight is metabolically inactive in fat stores.

Physical examination is vitally important and anthropometric measurements can be used to aid assessment of nutritional status.

DIETETIC MONITORING

Fluid balance

The importance of a daily accurate fluid balance chart detailing all fluid in (e.g. PN, other intravenous fluids, oral ontake) and all fluid out (e.g. urine, fistula, stoma, drains, diarrhoea) cannot be overemphasised. The clinical consequences of fluid overload include ankle, pulmonary and cardiac oedema, any of which may have significant deleterious effects on cardiac and respiratory function.

Fluid balance is calculated by assessment of total fluid input against total fluid excretion. A positive balance of about 500 ml is acceptable and will account for insensible losses from the lungs and through sweating. In warmer temperatures or with fever, insensible losses can increase considerably. This must be taken into consideration when calculating individual requirements.

Body weight and serum electrolytes, especially urea and sodium, are used as additional indicators as to the true state of a patient's hydration. Rapid fluctuations in daily weight will be due to fluid changes rather than to alterations in body mass (1 kg represents about 1 L of fluid). This enables a better understanding of the accuracy or otherwise of the fluid balance measurement. Urea and sodium are useful guides, since if both are high this may indicate dehydration, and if both are low this may indicate overhydration. However, the interpretation can be more difficult if, for example, the patient also has a high stoma output with large sodium losses that can lead to sodium depletion. In these situations correcting sodium losses by increasing sodium in the PN solution and/or using a side-arm on the PN with Hartmann's and titrating with output, as previously discussed, should correct the low sodium. If this is not successful, fluid balance issues need to be readdressed. Serum and urinary osmolality and sodium levels are also useful measurements. A high urinary sodium and high serum osmolality reflect an excessive intake, whereas low urinary sodium and osmolality reflect a low intake or high loss from another source, e.g. stoma.

Nitrogen balance

Nitrogen balance studies can be carried out on clinically stable patients. The majority of the nitrogen is excreted in the urine in the form of urea. The balance study involves an accurate 24 h urine collection, which is sent to the laboratory for urea and volume determination. From these figures urinary nitrogen can be calculated. To this figure an arbitrary 2–4 g of nitrogen is added to account for the losses of nitrogen from other sources, such as hair, skin, faeces and/or wounds. The final figure represents total nitrogen losses during the measured 24 h period. Nitrogen balance can be calculated from total nitrogen given via the PN (and orally) minus total nitrogen excreted. The main aim is for a zero to a positive balance of about 4 g.

If the balance is negative, the PN administered and the amount required need to be reassessed. There is an upper limit of nitrogen administration, deemed to be about 18 g, above which the nitrogen will not be assimilated into protein. The excess will be broken down and increase the urea produced. If the patient is in the catabolic stage of illness a positive nitrogen balance is unlikely to be achievable.

There are several practical problems associated with carrying out nitrogen balance studies. The main difficulty is collecting a full 24 h urine sample from patients who may not fully understand the importance and may forget, or feel that to leave collection pans behind them in the toilet for the nurse to deal with is causing unnecessary work. There are also problems with patients who have diarrhoea and void their bowels and bladder at the same time. In these situations a new collection needs to be started. The aim is initially for two to three collections a week and can be reduced to once a week. If a nitrogen balance result is negative it is worth repeating to check validity.

Urinalysis and blood sugar monitoring

Urinalysis is carried out to detect glucose overspill in the urine. This is performed by dipsticking the urine once a day. PN supplies a large amount of glucose to the body and, if insufficient endogenous insulin is produced, this will lead to high blood glucose levels. Excess glucose will be excreted by the kidneys. This means that energy is lost, and dehydration can occur due to osmotic diuresis. Certain clinical conditions predispose to glucose intolerance, e.g. pancreatitis, or when patients are still in the catabolic phase of their illness and insulin resistance occurs. When standard rather than tailored PN bags are supplied, a problem with excessive glucose calories may occur. In these situations close monitoring is essential.

When a positive urinalysis has been recorded, a blood sugar level is required to determine actual serum glucose. This can be carried out by fingerprick test strips and/or laboratory glucose level. Sliding-scale insulin is initiated by the doctor if the blood sugar levels are above 10 mmol/L. This enables more insulin units to be administered as and when the glucose level reaches a higher level. The insulin sliding-scale and blood sugar levels need to be monitored daily to make sure that the blood sugar levels are brought under control. The importance of monitoring blood sugar is discussed again in Chapter 10.

Trace element and vitamin monitoring

In Crohn's patients, longer-term patients in hospital and patients presenting with malnutrition, trace element and vitamin screening is an essential part of their care. The policy for which trace elements and vitamins need screening will vary from hospital to hospital. The following are generally measured: zinc, magnesium, manganese, copper, selenium, iron, ferritin; and vitamins A, E, D, B_{12}, thiamin, riboflavin and pyridoxine. Zinc, magnesium and haemoglobin are monitored weekly in stable patients. The other trace elements and vitamins are monitored 3-monthly in longer-term patients.

NUTRITIONAL COMPLICATIONS OF PN

Refeeding syndrome

Malnourished patients and other vulnerable patients, such as alcoholics and patients on long-term diuretics or antacids, are at a greater risk of developing 'refeeding syndrome' (Solomon & Kirby 1990). Refeeding syndrome is defined as severe fluid and electrolyte shifts that give rise to altered biochemical levels, which in turn lead to cardiac, respiratory, hepatic, renal, GI tract, neuromuscular and haematological problems. The consequences are low phosphate, potassium, magnesium, altered glucose metabolism, vitamin deficiency and fluid balance abnormalities. The more immediate effects of low potassium, phosphate and magnesium are cardiac arrhythmias, which can lead to cardiac arrest. It is therefore recommended that the levels of these electrolytes are checked and corrected *before* starting PN and monitored daily for at least 7–10 days in at-risk patients.

Electrolyte swings can also occur once PN has started. In starvation, despite body depletion, serum electrolyte concentrations can appear normal owing to alterations in renal excretion. During refeeding there is a switch in metabolism, with carbohydrate repletion and increased insulin production. This leads to an increase in the uptake of glucose, phosphorus, potassium, and water into the cells, thereby leading to severe extracellular depletion of electrolytes. At-risk patients should also be given a large dose of thiamin before PN is commenced, as thiamin levels may be depleted (Solomon & Kirby 1990) (e.g. Pabrinex containing 250 mg/dose thiamin or Multibionta containing 50 mg/dose).

Thiamin plays an essential role in carbohydrate metabolism. Wernicke's encephalopathy, an acute confusional state, can be precipitated by feeding with carbohydrate in vitamin B-depleted patients. The treatment is thiamin repletion, 50 mg i.v. for the first 3 days. Thereafter if the patient is on PN thiamin will be-provided as part of the vitamin preparation, e.g. Cernevit 3.5 mg thiamin, or Multibionta 50 mg, or Solivito 3.2 mg; otherwise an oral dose of 100 mg daily until the patient is re-established onto a balanced diet. Calorie delivery should initially be slower than in patients not at risk, for example roughly half of the calories required. This should be increased to a normal rate after the first 24 h. In practical terms this could mean starting with one bag over 2 days and then reverting to the normal infusion of one bag per day.

Overfeeding

Overfeeding can be a problem in situations where standard bags are used universally and patients receive a larger amount of total calories and nitrogen than they need.

Effects of overfeeding calories

The most immediate effect of giving excess carbohydrate to a patient who is being ventilated or who has low pulmonary reserve is to increase the amount of oxygen consumed and carbon dioxide produced. This can potentially tip a patient into respiratory failure. High carbohydrate administration may prevent the weaning of a patient from a ventilator (Elwyn 1993). In ventilated patients this will be shown by increased carbon dioxide retention and a faster respiratory rate.

Long-term side-effects of excessive carbohydrate and/or fat include fatty liver and liver dysfunction, evidenced by jaundice and high levels of liver enzymes (Wolfe et al 1980). Lipogenesis and fluid and fat gain, rather than lean body mass, also occur. However, standard bags rarely provide more than 2500 kcal, of which approximately 50% of energy comes from lipid and 50% from glucose. A maximum glucose oxidation has been established, above which glucose cannot be metabolised. This rate is 4–7 mg/kg/min/day (Todorovick & Micklewright 1997), which translates to about 1600 kcal/day for a 70 kg man. Similarly, there is a maximum rate for lipid infusion of 2–5 g/kg/day in adults. For a 70 kg patient this represents 1575 kcal/day. The standard bag mentioned here falls well within these constraints. Lipid clearance should be checked, particularly in patients who are critically ill, those with liver and/or renal failure, and in patients with pancreatitis. This is carried out by monitoring baseline triglycerides (now also known as triacylglycerol) and cholesterol levels, and then weekly triglycerides. Triglyceride levels should always be checked in patients whose blood is recorded as 'lipaemic'. Plasma triglyceride levels should be checked several hours after the infusion is complete and should never be taken from the PN line owing to problems of contamination.

In the event of an elevated triglyceride level the lipid provided may need to be reduced accordingly, or even removed for a couple of days a week, to reduce the triglyceride levels and the liver enzymes. This is discussed in more detail in the section *Manipulations in response to high liver enzymes*.

Effects of overfeeding nitrogen

Excess nitrogen to requirements will cause increased oxygen consumption and carbon dioxide production during metabolism. Serum urea will rise as the extra nitrogen puts a strain on the kidneys. This is especially important in patients with renal insufficiency. Most sources agree that levels about 18 g nitrogen/day will not be used efficiently and are therefore not justified. A positive nitrogen balance of 4–6 g nitrogen/day is ideal, but this can only be achieved in a stable anabolic patient. It is not possible to obtain a positive balance in the early stages of injury and providing excessive nitrogen to offset this will cause more harm than good.

Manipulations in response to high liver enzymes

Standard bags of PN can be used for most patients providing adequate monitoring takes place. If it is found that a patient develops respiratory problems or has raised triglyceride levels associated with the PN, then steps need to be taken to reduce the use of glucose and lipid, respectively.

Cyclical PN involves increasing the rate of infusion so as to deliver the PN bag over a shorter time. This can improve liver function tests (LFTs), as the liver is given a break from high levels of circulating glucose and lipid. This also gives the patient time away from her drip stand and increases the opportunity of mobility. Cyclical PN often boosts morale and enables more flexible family contact, and patients living nearby may even be able to go home for part of the day. If the patient is able to take small amounts of fluid and/or food by mouth this will also aid the reduction of LFTs by stimulation. The liver usually receives 'first pass' of nutrients, which stimulates gall bladder contraction and produces bile salts rather than leading to an accumulation of biliary sludge. However, even if the patient is strictly nil by mouth, a few hours' rest from PN can be of benefit to the liver (Thomas 1994).

Another useful manipulation is the theoretical benefit of a mixture of lipid which contains some medium chain triglycerides (MCT) instead of the more usual use of 100% long chain triglycerides (LCT). MCT is more rapidly oxidised than LCT, giving rise to faster energy production with less lipid deposition (Dennison et al 1988). It is also useful for stressed patients who are better able to metabolise MCT/LCT lipid than LCT alone (Thomas 1994).

If liver function levels remain high after the above alterations to the PN, then the last resort is to remove the lipid altogether. However, to prevent essential fatty acid deficiency lipid needs to be given twice a week (Thomas 1994). These bags can be spaced out in the week. Reducing the total number of calories given will also help to lower the LFTs.

Short bowel syndrome

Short bowel syndrome is defined as less than 150 cm of functioning small bowel. This may be the result of Crohn's or Hirschsprung's disease, or resection of the bowel for tumour removal or infarction. Nutritional problems include dehydration and electrolyte imbalance, especially sodium, magnesium and zinc. Other problems include malabsorption of macro- and micro-nutrients and rapid transit time.

The precise length and section of remaining gut is important information. The ileum is the specific site for vitamin B_{12} absorption. If this section has been resected, then vitamin B_{12} injections will be required 3-monthly and serum levels will need to be monitored on a regular basis.

Although many of these patients may require PN for life, those with approximately 200 cm of small bowel remaining have a limited working capacity and time will be required for full adaptation of the remaining small bowel. The problems involved in weaning such patients from PN are discussed below.

WEANING FROM PN

Once a patient has been on PN for a few days and is biochemically stable, the number of hours the PN is infused over can be reduced. The exceptions to this would be:

- Patients on intensive care (ICU) where hourly fluid monitoring occurs and background infusions are best kept evenly distributed over the day.
- Patients with congestive cardiac failure who are unlikely to cope well with large fluid intakes.
- Patients with large losses from the GI tract who would dehydrate if no i.v. fluid was given, e.g. stoma, fistula, nasogastric losses.
- Patients with unstable electrolytes who would benefit from a 24 h infusion, particularly those with a high sodium and potassium requirement.
- Patients at risk of developing pulmonary oedema where an even distribution of fluid is more likely to keep them in status quo.
- Patients with unstable blood sugars.

For other patients, PN can be gradually reduced from 24 h to 20, 16 and then 12 h as tolerated. This enables greater flexibility of movement without the encumbrance of the infusion and drip stand. When the PN line is not in use care must be taken that the i.v. access does not become blocked (for details of how to care for a line to prevent occlusion, see Ch. 7).

If a patient has been requiring sliding-scale insulin to keep her blood glucose within the normal range whilst on PN, then this must be stopped once the patient comes off PN or hypoglycaemia can result. It is currently recommended that the infusion rate of PN is halved for the last hour on PN in order to get the body used to a lower glucose load and reduce endogenous production of insulin. However, there is evidence in both adults and children that abrupt discontinuation of PN is well tolerated in stable patients (Werlin et al 1994). Other investigators have shown that the islet cells in the pancreas are able to respond within minutes to changes in the level of glucose infused (Krzywda et al 1993). Even so, there is clearly a group of patients in whom more care should be taken: children under 3 years, patients on insulin, and patients who have demonstrated swings in their blood glucose control.

Weaning a patient from total PN support to an enteral diet needs to be taken by stages. A patient cannot be expected to revert to a normal diet as soon as clinically indicated, especially if she has not eaten for a period of more than 1–2 weeks. The cells lining the GI tract have a fast turnover rate, and are quick to lose the surface microvilli that play a key function in the absorption of nutrients. Enzyme production is also reduced when the gut is not in use. Initially there may be a degree of malabsorption until the absorptive surface increases and the enzymes are once again fully functional.

PN has been shown to delay gastric emptying in normal healthy male subjects fed less than half of their total basal energy requirements. This may explain why patients on PN have reduced appetites and why it can be difficult for some patients to increase their voluntary food intake (Bursztein-De Myttenaere et al 1994). PN suppresses appetite proportionally to the amount of energy and nitrogen provided. However, some workers have found that glucose has a greater appetite-suppressant effect than lipid (Gil et al 1991). Appetite will not improve overnight as it takes a number of days before the appetite-suppressing effect of PN has disappeared. Cyclical PN has not been found to alleviate this problem as it is likely to be the total number of calories administered, in particular lipid calories, that affects appetite (Opara et al 1995). This is where a 48 h bag can be useful, as discussed below.

Other factors affecting appetite include primary disease, e.g. cancer, chronic inflammatory bowel disease, poor mobility, pain, pyrexia, nausea and vomiting, and depression. The smell of the PN can also be off-putting and patients sometimes develop a metallic taste that may be associated with the lipid fraction of the PN mixture. This taste sensation can be alleviated by eating citrus fruits and/or pineapple, but the taste change will often not resolve until the PN has stopped. All these factors lead to a poor food intake and patients require a lot of encouragement from the nurse, dietitian, relatives and friends involved in their care.

The normal weaning process from PN is to take sips of water, gradually increasing to clear fluids, then onto free fluids as tolerated. Diet is then introduced as soup and puddings, progressing to main courses, taking into account any therapeutic dietary manipulations required. Patients who have received PN over prolonged periods may experience pain and gastric disturbances once an enteral diet is introduced, which is both distressing and demoralising. Food is encouraged 'little and often' to help the patient to build up an appetite.

As the enteral diet increases it is important to keep accurate daily fluid and food record charts for assessment by the dietitian. Enteral nutritional supplements can also be encouraged in most cases to enhance the patient's calorie and protein intake. Once a patient manages approximately half of her daily calorie requirement via the enteral route, a 48 h bag of PN can be administered. The rationale behind this is to enable the patient time to increase her oral intake whilst still benefiting from partial parenteral support. The use of a 48 h bag may then be reviewed alongside the food record chart. When the NST are confident that the patient is tolerating an adequate oral intake, PN can be discontinued. The central venous access device by which the PN has been administered normally remains in position for a few more days to ensure the patient has clearly demonstrated her ability to tolerate an adequate enteral diet. However, if energy intake falls, nutritional supplements are encouraged.

On the ICU, or in cases where patients are unable or unwilling to take sufficient food orally, a nasogastric feed can be commenced as a method of weaning from a more invasive form of feeding to a more physiologically normal route.

Weaning the patient with short bowel syndrome from PN

Weaning such patients from PN takes time and consideration for adequate fluid replacement and requires a sound knowledge of specific nutrient deficiencies. Initially stoma outputs can be high and it is often difficult to gauge the amount a patient is actually absorbing from her diet. In this instance regular vitamin and trace element analysis is essential, as described earlier.

One method of reducing stoma output is to restrict the intake of hypotonic fluids, e.g. tea, coffee, water and squash, to 500–700 ml/day, and to encourage small, frequent meals with added salt, with drinks taken between meals rather than at meals. Oral rehydration therapy is encouraged, e.g. World Health Organisation (WHO) solution as often as required, up to 2 L/day, depending on the patient's hydration state. Indications of dehydration are discussed in Chapter 7 and include dark urine, poor urine output, thirst, and dry lips and skin.

CONCLUSION

This chapter has discussed dietetic aspects of PN. The role of EN cannot be overstated – all EN routes should have been thoroughly investigated before resorting to PN. However, if the gut is non-functioning or inaccessible for more than a week, then PN is the remaining choice. PN is not normally considered to be of benefit unless it is required for more than 7–10 days. PN should not be considered as an emergency procedure in adult patients. In malnourished patients short-term PN (required for less than 7 days) can be administered via a peripheral cannula. For shorter periods of time the risk of inserting a central line outweighs the benefit gained.

Dietetic assessment needs to take into account relevant past medical history, current presenting complaint including liver/renal impairment, and any large fluid outputs, e.g. stoma losses. Calorie, nitrogen, fluid and electrolyte requirements are then assessed based on gender, current weight, temperature, activity level and changing clinical condition.

In general standard bags of PN are used; so long as adequate monitoring is undertaken, these should be suitable for most patients. However, there are circumstances when more individualised bags are required, for example for fluid and electrolyte alterations, and where there is liver and renal impairment.

Dietetic monitoring includes a detailed examination of the daily fluid balance, body weight, electrolytes and liver function tests, urinalysis, nitrogen balance calculations, urine electrolytes and any oral intake. From this information and any developments from a medical and nursing perspective the PN mixture and the daily plan can be altered as necessary. Potential nutritional complications to be aware of include the refeeding syndrome, overfeeding, and deranged liver function.

Once a patient has been established on PN and is haemodynamically and biochemically stable, the infusion rate can be increased to allow time free of PN and the drip stand. This tends to increase patient mobility and raise morale. It is normally recommended that the infusion rate is halved the hour before the PN is stopped to allow the patient time to adapt to a lower glucose infusion.

Weaning a patient off PN onto oral diet needs to be taken by stages and may involve the introduction of a 48 h bag of PN in order to reduce total calorie delivery whilst encouraging oral intake. It is important to start weaning a patient as soon as possible from PN so that the complications alluded to in this chapter are minimised.

REFERENCES

Bursztein-De Myttenaere S, Gil KM, Heymsfield SB 1994 Gastric emptying in humans: influence of different regimens of parenteral nutrition. American Journal Clinical Nutrition 60:244–248

Dennison R, Ball M, Hando LJ, Crowe PJ, Watkins RM, Kettlewell M 1988 Total parenteral nutrition using conventional and medium chain triglycerides: effect on liver function tests, complement, and nitrogen balance. Journal of Parenteral and Enteral Nutrition 12:15 19

Elwyn DH 1993 Carbohydrate metabolism and requirements for nutritional support: part III. Nutrition 9(3):255–267

Garrow JS 1981 Treat obesity seriously: a clinical manual. Churchill Livingstone, Edinburgh, pp 27–29

Gil KM, Skeie B, Kvetan V, Ashkenazi J, Friedman MI 1991 Parenteral nutrition and oral intake: effect of glucose and fat infusions. Journal of Parenteral and Enteral Nutrition 15:426–432

Krzywda EA, Andris DA, Whipple JK 1993 Glucose response to abrupt initiation and discontinuation of total parenteral nutrition. Journal of Parenteral and Enteral Nutrition 17:64–67

Lee HA 1974 Composition of some body external secretions. In: Parenteral nutrition in acute metabolic illness, table VI, p 101. Academic Press, London

Opara EI, Meguid MM, Yang ZJ, Chai JK, Veerabagu M 1995 Tumor necrosis factor-α and total parenteral nutrition-induced anorexia. Surgery 118:756–762

Solomon SM, Kirby DF, 1990 The refeeding syndrome: a review. Journal of Parenteral and Enteral Nutrition 14:90–97

Todorovick VE, Micklewright A 1997 A pocket guide to clinical nutrition. British Dietetic Association, Birmingham, section 3.1

Thomas 1994 Parenteral nutrition. In: Manual of dietetic practice. Blackwell, Oxford, ch 15, p 80

Werlin SL, Wyatt D, Camitta B 1994 Effect of abrupt discontinuation of high glucose infusion rates during parenteral nutrition. Journal of Pediatrics 124:441–444

Wolfe RR, O'Donnell TF, Store MD, Richmond DA, Burke JF 1980 Investigation of factors determining the optimal glucose infusion rate in total parenteral nutrition. Metabolism 79:897–900

9

Complications

Louise Sherliker

Introduction
Complications related to central venous
  catheters

Complications related to equipment
Conclusion

INTRODUCTION

This chapter analyses the complications associated with parenteral nutrition (PN). The first part of the chapter concentrates on catheter-related complications and includes helpful advice about diagnosis, prevention and management of these problems. The next section examines mechanical complications of PN. Finally, complications related to the patient, including consideration of metabolic complications, are analysed.

COMPLICATIONS RELATED TO CENTRAL VENOUS CATHETERS

Success in the use of indwelling central venous catheters (cvcs) to administer PN has been reported for almost two decades. This progress has led to further developments in the types of catheters used, and the methods of their placement. The complications related to the insertion and type of catheter used are discussed in other chapters; however, the most commonly described complications associated with cvcs are catheter-related sepsis, catheter occlusions, haemorrhage, severance, pneumothorax and air embolism. All of these complications will be discussed in turn, and directions in the management of these problems will be explored.

Catheter-related sepsis

Catheter related sepsis is the most common type of catheter complication (Tolar & Gould 1996). The catheter infection rate of a Unit can be influenced by a range of factors from type of device and dressing technique, to education of staff and patients. It is important therefore that strategies to prevent infections are observed not only from a single perspective, but also placed in a broad context. It is therefore important that potential site and diagnosis of infection are observed in greater detail.

Sites of infection

Patients are primarily prone to colonisation of microorganisms on the surface of the skin. These can invade the insertion wound either at the time of insertion or in following days, resulting in a local infection or generalised septicaemia. It is believed that catheters with subcutaneous Dacron cuffs, which eventually fibrose into the surrounding tissue, for example Hickman catheters, provide a mechanical barrier to these invading organisms; this is reflected by their lower rates of infections (Maki 1991).

Another potential site for infection is the catheter hub, and it is thought that in longer-term devices this site may pose the greatest threat to infection. Contamination of infusion fluid remains a further potential risk. Microorganisms can be easily introduced during the preparation and administration of intravenous drugs or solutions either at the hospital site or during manufacture. Many studies have indicated that the choice of a venous access device may also have an impact on infection rates. Apart from the presence of a Dacron cuff as mentioned previously, some research has suggested that multilumen catheters are associated with higher infection rates in comparison to single-lumen catheters, whereas some studies suggest that certain materials used in manufacture of central catheters are preferable to others. However, research studies into the adherence of microorganisms to the inside of the catheter have produced conflicting results. The length of time a catheter has been in place may also influence infection rates, since it is thought that the longer the catheter is in situ the more susceptible it is to infection. Some studies advocate the removal or replacement of lines after certain time periods. Cunha (1995) suggests that non-dwelling lines should be replaced on a basis that relates to the colonisation time of catheters, which has shown to be approximately 7 days.

Insertion technique and experience in this speciality may also be a contributing factor that may influence infection rates. In Oxford, the employment of a clinical nurse specialist to insert cvcs has reduced infection rates in tunnelled feeding lines to less than 1% (Hamilton 1993).

Diagnosis

Maki (1991) explains that septicaemia due to catheter infection may not always be easy to distinguish from other infections, for example a urinary tract infection. It is therefore important that blood cultures are taken at any sign of infection, even if the infection appears not to be related to the catheter, and especially if there appears to be no focus of infection. Blood cultures should be drawn from the catheter and a peripheral vein. This is because blood cultures drawn from an infected catheter usually contain a ten times greater concentration of organisms.

The clinical signs in a patient with a catheter-related sepsis may vary from mild to extreme. The majority of patients, apart from those who are immunosuppressed, will experience a rise in temperature. The heart rate may also rise, and the patient may feel shivery, hot, achy and unwell. If the sepsis is related to the insertion site the area may look red, inflamed and feel sore. In addition there may be a purulent discharge. If the patient has a skin-tunnelled catheter, which is common in those patients receiving long-term PN, the patient may experience a red 'tracking' from the exit site of the catheter towards the incision site near the collar bone. In all cases, the patient must be educated to recognise the signs of infection and act accordingly. If the patient feels unwell and experiences a sudden rise in temperature he must be observed closely, since septic shock is a potential result, whereupon the patient will need emergency support and antibiotics.

Prevention

The prevention of sepsis due to central venous catheterisation must be a priority in patient care for any healthcare professional involved in the management of intravenous therapy. This importance is emphasised further if the patient is immunocompromised, since negligence in this area could easily prove fatal. In any area, the use of research-based protocols that define procedures and lead to uniformity of care must be an imperative. However, a protocol must be user friendly and reflect the consensus opinion of the team. It must also be a 'working' protocol that is not laid down in stone, but provides a basis for regular assessment and evaluation and is flexible enough to respond to new evidence and innovations.

The care of cvcs is becoming more technical and specialised, with the development of many associated products ranging from dressings to access devices. Research studies evaluating procedures and products have historically been small and inconclusive, leading to confusion and variance in practice. It is therefore important for the healthcare professional not only to analyse critically data and findings, but also to produce a protocol that is in keeping with the environment, culture and resources of her workplace, and most importantly with philosophy of care.

The following sections do not provide a black and white plan of how to prevent and care for the associated complications of central lines, but analyse critically directions of care, providing information and support to enable the reader to make informed choices about strategies for care.

Caring for the central line. Since a high proportion of catheter-related sepsis is a direct result of cutaneous microorganisms, it is important that an appropriate cleansing solution and dressing is used. The problem with this statement is that there is a huge divergence in opinion in what is deemed to be 'appropriate'. Past studies that analyse the efficacy of cleansing solutions and dressings often fail to arrive at firm conclusions, or if a conclusion is made there is often another study offering conflicting advice. This is mainly due to the fact that infection rates and catheter care are influenced by many variables. For example, no one hospital ward is identical – one area may wear sterile gloves, another may have different insertion practices, another may have different antibiotic protocols, or use different catheters. Hence, the moral of the story is: analyse the evidence, form a protocol that is relevant to your area, implement the protocol, and then review and evaluate regularly, and change as required. The following sections will review some of the current practices for catheter care.

Cleansing solutions. A study by Maki et al (1991) compared the efficacy of three solutions, 70% alcohol, 10% povidone-iodine and 2% aqueous chlorhexidine, used in the prevention of catheter-related sepsis. They concluded that the use of 2% chlorhexidine made significant reductions in the incidence of catheter infections. However, it has been suggested (Perry & Leaper 1994) that chlorhexidine, which is a more active agent against Gram-positive than Gram-negative infections, should be used for short-term catheter care, whereas povidone-iodine, which has a broader antibacterial spectrum, should be used for long-term catheter care. Hydrogen peroxide has been used in the past to assist in the removal of exudate, but there is little evidence indicating its effectiveness in this area. Normal saline (sodium chloride 0.9%), which is often a solution of choice for wound cleaning, is thought not to be sufficiently effective in comparison to antiseptic solutions, especially considering that patients who require this level of intervention and intravenous support are often deemed to be at a higher risk of infection.

Maki & McCormack (1987) studied the use of defatting catheter insertion sites to reduce infection. Acetone was used to remove microorganisms from lipids on the skin surface, but to no significant effect. Any new solution to be used on a catheter should be checked against manufacturer's recommendations, since some solutions may be contraindicated and have a negative effect on the catheter material.

Dressings. At this present time there are two schools of thought as to which dressing to use for a cvc. The first school advocates the traditional method of gauze and tape. The second school advocates the use of transparent polyurethane (vapour permeable) film dressings.

A gauze dressing will require changing every 24–48 h, depending on factors such as the age of the line and leakage from the insertion site. Gauze dressings, which are significantly cheaper, are thought to be easier for patients to handle; this may be important in a unit promoting self-care. However, they are not waterproof and will need to be changed immediately that the dressing becomes wet, for example following a shower or a bath.

There has been much controversy over the past few years surrounding the safety and effectiveness of transparent dressings in the short and long term. Some studies suggest that using transparent dressings is comparable in terms of catheter-related sepsis rates to gauze dressings, owing to the reduction in frequency of changing the dressing, and hence the reduced likelihood of introducing microorganisms (Lawson et al. 1986). The advantages of transparent sterile dressings are that they allow the site to be continually inspected, they are waterproof, allow secure fixation and are impervious to bacteria. However, concern in the past has focused upon whether collection of moisture under the dressing, combined with the warm environment, leads to an increase in cutaneous colonisation and therefore infection (Hoffmann et al 1992).

Brandt et al (1996), in comparing daily gauze dressings with transparent dressings in bone marrow transplant recipients, concluded that there was no statistical difference between the two types of dressings. However, this group of patients found the transparent dressings comfortable, and they were found to be more cost-effective in relation to the gauze dressings. Patient preference and skin tolerance will undoubtedly have a contributory influence in decision making about these dressings.

Occlusions

An occlusion of a central venous catheter is usually detected when a fluid cannot be infused or blood cannot be withdrawn from the catheter. Occlusion of cvcs may be due to a variety of reasons from mechanical obstruction to thrombosis, lipid deposits or the precipitation of drugs. This section will analyse the problems associated with occlusion of lines from diagnosis to prevention, and to resolution and evaluation.

Diagnosis

It is important that the nature of the occlusion is determined prior to attempting to restore patency of the lumen. The first step is to examine the catheter visually for kinking, clamping or any other mechanical obstruction. If nothing is apparent, radiological examination may be required. An X-ray can determine the position of the catheter tip, while injecting radio-opaque dye into the catheter can verify if there is an obstruction and verify its location. This will be impossible in completely blocked catheters, which will not allow any fluid to be injected, but is useful in partially blocked catheters, including those that will allow fluid to be infused, but will not allow blood to be withdrawn. Care must be taken at all times so that no undue pressure is exerted, leading to damage of the catheter in the form of a rupture, or that clots are flushed into the patient.

One of the most common reasons for catheter occlusion is the formation of a thrombus or clot. A thrombus may be seen as a natural response to the presence of a foreign body within the system. This results in the utilisation of platelets and the formation of a fibrin 'flap', usually observed at the tip of the catheter. Clinically, this may initially be seen as the inability to withdraw blood from the catheter despite the catheter allowing the infusion of fluid. Eventually the fibrin flap may become a 'plug', and the catheter will become completely occluded (Fig. 9.1). A clinically significant major venous thrombosis has been reported in up to 5% of patients receiving cvcs. An obstruction such as this may actually be asymptomatic and only discovered if a new line requires insertion. However, the patient may feel pain and swelling of the neck and arm. This would be indicative of this type of complication and an ultrasound or venogram of the area would be required.

Clots may also form if blood products are administered very slowly via

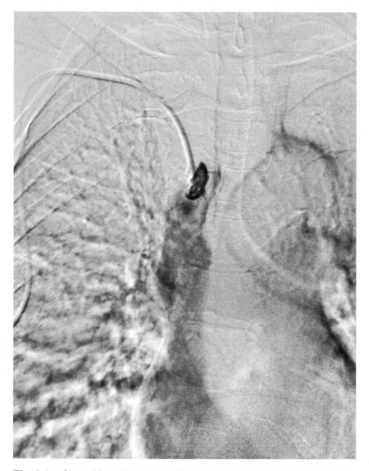

Fig. 9.1 Chest X-ray demonstrating, with the use of contrast medium, the fibrin flap occluding the cvc used for PN.

the catheter, resulting in coagulation, or if blood back-flows from the vein into the catheter. A second reason for catheter occlusion is the formation of lipid deposits within the lumen of the PN catheter. In this situation the catheter can perform sluggishly over a period of 2–3 days before becoming completely occluded.

Prevention

Catheter patency is a priority when caring for patients with central venous lines. Flushing of the catheter is essential in the prevention of complications. This is done by inserting into the catheter a solution, usually containing an anticoagulant, at the end of an infusion, between infusions, after the removal of blood, or when the catheter is not required for a period of time.

Flushing a catheter with sodium chloride (0.9%), followed by a solution of heparin, is the recommended technique to maintain patency. However, as Kelly et al (1992) explain, there is much controversy over the volume and dose of heparin administered, as well as the frequency of flushing. The controversy appears to lie in the fact that too much flushing of a catheter heightens the potential for microorganisms to be introduced, whereas too little flushing is linked with increased potential for thrombotic complications, which are associated with catheter sepsis (Raad et al 1994). Kelly et al (1992), after reviewing flushing protocols in the USA, researched the implementation of a protocol which advised that long-term cvcs should be flushed weekly with 5 ml of 10 u/ml heparin and saline, and this is what is recommended on the Haematology Unit in Oxford. However, as with controversies surrounding other techniques, the most important advice is that a protocol is established, implemented, and then its effectiveness reviewed on a regular basis.

Documentation of complications is essential, and it is highly important that the complications are communicated between health professionals, whether they are community or hospital based. Education of patients, carers and other healthcare professionals is vital in the provision of optimum catheter care. Teaching a patient or relative to flush their own catheter helps to involve them in their treatment, but also gives the patient a degree of control and responsibility, which is often lost in the fight to restore health. The employment of a community intravenous nurse specialist in certain areas of the UK not only provides the link with community care, but also provides education, training and support to both healthcare professionals and patients receiving home PN (HPN), which ultimately can lead to longer periods at home for the patient.

Unblocking a catheter

Urokinase and streptokinase are the thrombolytics commonly used to dissolve clots that have formed in catheters. However, streptokinase has a higher incidence of anaphylactic reactions, and therefore urokinase tends to be the treatment of choice.

If a clot is suspected or diagnosed within the lumen, a solution of urokinase should be administered. A suggested dilution is: urokinase 5000 iu diluted in 3 ml of 0.9% sodium chloride. The appropriate volume, e.g. the indwelling volume of the catheter lumen, should be slowly injected into the catheter using a 'push–pull' action in order that the drug is mixed as much as possible within the lumen.

The catheter should then be clamped and left for 2–3 h. After this time the clot will hopefully have been dispersed, and should be carefully withdrawn from the catheter. If the catheter is still occluded, then the process can be repeated a further time for a longer period, and some centres do promote the use of a urokinase infusion (Haire et al 1990). However, if the patient is already at risk from bleeding, for example a patient with an abnormal platelet count, then caution is advised. Prolonged and untreatable blockage of a catheter will inevitably lead to removal. In some centres physicians advise the prophylactic use of low-dose warfarin to prevent these complications.

Other occlusions

Patients receiving PN formulations are prone to catheter occlusion due to the build-up of lipid material within the catheter lumen. This may be difficult to distinguish from a thrombosis, but it usually follows a pattern of increasing difficulty in being able to flush the catheter over a period of time, owing to the formation of a lipid 'sludge'. The catheter must therefore be flushed vigorously with normal saline on a daily basis, and prior to connection of a new infusion set. If it is felt that the catheter is gradually becoming occluded, it is often advisable to use urokinase before the lumen becomes totally occluded.

In the event that urokinase is not effective it can often be assumed that, given the behaviour of the catheter, the cause of the occlusion is lipid deposits within the catheter. The use of 70% ethanol solution, administered with extreme caution, to the affected lumen will aid in dissolving the lipid material. The catheter should then be flushed vigorously with sodium chloride.

Other occlusions may be due to the kinking of the catheter in the vein, or the tip of the catheter lying against the vein wall and hence inhibiting the clear flow of fluid. In both cases a change in the position of the patient is advised, and is particularly helpful if withdrawal of blood from the catheter is required. Tilting the patient's head backwards may help to move the catheter away from the vessel wall, along with lying on one side or raising arms upwards and engaging in deep inspirations. It is obviously impractical for the patient to perform these manoeuvres over a long period of time, and therefore manipulation of the line under X-ray guidance may be necessary.

Haemorrhage

Haemorrhage around the site can occur during or immediately post insertion, or due to trauma, for example in the case of inadvertently pulling the line. Post cvc insertion, a patient should be observed closely for haemorrhage by performing their vital signs regularly. The frequency of recording observations will depend upon local guidelines, and will be affected by factors such as whether the patient received a general anaesthetic or mild sedation.

A normal clotting profile is essential for the safe insertion of a cvc. In a small group of patients it may be necessary to provide alternative methods of stabilising the patient's clotting profile using blood products. If a patient is thrombocytopaenic he may require a platelet transfusion prior to insertion of the catheter.

Slight bleeding around the site of catheter insertion is not uncommon. A pressure dressing may be applied to the site, which will control bleeding to a certain extent. Bleeding due to trauma of the line is a rare, serious complication. However, a sterile dressing should be applied, and the patient instructed to ensure that the line is securely fastened to prevent further potential trauma.

Severance

Any rupture, damage or leakage from the catheter must be acted upon immediately to prevent blood loss or an air embolism forming. The catheter should be clamped proximal to the damaged area or close to the exit site. A sterile dressing should be applied to the affected area. It is important that patients are informed of this potentially serious problem, and are aware of what action to take in the event of this occuring. Each hospital area should have a sterile repair kit available for this emergency, which should correspond to the manufacturer of the catheter in situ.

The instructions will vary depending on the catheter manufacturer, e.g. either an adhesive or non-adhesive method. It is therefore important that the healthcare professional has experience or fully reads the instructions before using the repair kit.

Pneumothorax

Pneumothorax is a complication associated with the insertion of cvcs via the neck and chest. It is thought that the incidence of this problem may increase if the patient is thin and malnourished, possibly because there is less intervening fat and muscle deposit between the lung wall and the vein. Pneumothorax is also more prevalent in patients with respiratory disease or those requiring artificial ventilation, causing the lungs to become hyperinflated.

If the pneumothorax occurs at the time of line insertion the patient may experience sharp chest pain, or shoulder tip pain and shortness of breath, and may cough due to pleuritic irritation. The severity of these symptoms is dependent on the size of the pneumothorax. However, if the patient is sedated at the time of insertion, these symptoms may be masked, and the pneumothorax may only be detected on a chest X-ray. It is therefore essential that a chest X-ray is performed immediately post insertion to rule out the presence of this complication, plus determining that the catheter is in the correct position. A pneumothorax at the time of line insertion is usually small in nature, and will normally not require intervention in the form of a chest drain. If a chest drain is inserted it is usually only required for 2–3 days, at which time there is spontaneous resolution of the air leak. A small pneumothorax should resolve within 2–5 days, and should not require any intervention, although regular monitoring through chest X-rays is suggested. The patient will exhibit few symptoms during this period. The most common symptom is pleuritic chest discomfort that may radiate to the shoulder or the back.

Although the peak incidence for a pneumothorax to occur is around the time of insertion, it is also possible that it may develop up to a few days post insertion. This delayed occurrence is typically related to difficult line insertions requiring multiple attempts to locate the subclavian vein with the insertion needle. This delayed response is also characterised by sudden chest or back pain often associated with a non-productive but irritable cough. An immediate chest X-ray will be required to determine the absence of a pneumothorax and the position of the cvc.

Air embolism

An air embolism is a potentially fatal complication of central venous cannulation. It may occur if the intravenous tubing becomes detached from the end of the catheter, leading to inspiration of air. It is estimated that only 200 ml of air, which can easily be passed through a catheter in just a few seconds, can lead to death. The majority of cvcs today have some sort of device to prevent this complication, either a clamp proximal to the patient, or a valve at the tip of the catheter to prevent blood from back-flowing or air from entering. It is, however, advisable to teach healthcare professionals and patients to keep the clamps in the closed position whenever the catheter is not being used.

If the patient is in distress due to an air embolism he will become dyspnoeic, experience chest pain, have an increased respiratory rate, become tachycardic, and may also be cyanosed. Potentially this problem could lead to cardiac arrest. If any of the above symptoms occur due to a suspected potential air embolism, the catheter should be clamped immediately and the patient should be placed on his left side with his head tipped down. This will enable air to be trapped in the right atrium or ventricle, allowing pulmonary outflow to continue, without the air causing a significant obstruction. The patient will then require direct aspiration of the air from the right side of the heart.

COMPLICATIONS RELATED TO EQUIPMENT

Problems with infusion pump devices

The use of an infusion pump is a well-recognised safety measure to prevent the associated problems related to normal gravity drips. Parenteral nutrition often requires a large amount of fluid to be infused over a long period of time. An infusion pump will enable the fluid to be infused at a constant rate, and will prevent problems like excessive fluid being infused too quickly or the catheter becoming occluded, both of which can have potentially serious and life-threatening effects on the patient.

However, infusion pumps, if not used correctly by trained staff, can also lead to potentially serious complications, and it is important that these points are considered:

- Never use an infusion pump unless you are familiar with, or have been trained to operate the machine.
- Ensure the infusion pump has an audible alarm to detect an air embolism.
- Ensure the infusion pump has an audible alarm to detect an occlusion, and is set to a recognised pressure setting. This is important so that unwanted pressure on the catheter is detected quickly, and is not allowed to build up to a high level before it is detected. This could lead to damage of the catheter and potential build up of fluid causing back pressure.
- Ensure that the infusion pump is clean before using.
- If the infusion pump is battery maintained and the patient wishes to mobilise, then ensure the pump is fully charged before use or there is access to an electric socket.
- If any of the above problems necessitate a long period where the infusion is not being administered, the infusion will need to be disconnected and flushed so that the line does not occlude.

Split or damaged bags

If a bag containing PN is seen to be damaged or split, causing leakage of the fluid, then it must be discarded. The infusion should be disconnected immediately. Parenteral nutrition is an excellent medium for potential growth of microorganisms. It is therefore prepared under strict aseptic guidelines, and any break in the enclosed sterile system will inevitably lead to sepsis.

Complications related to the patient

The safe administration of PN relies upon knowledge of potential metabolic complications of the therapy. This part of the chapter examines these complications in relation to the effects upon the organs and systems of the body, but also in relation to how the individual feels or reacts if these complications occur.

Glucose intolerance

Grant (1992) explains that adult patients can usually tolerate correctly calculated doses of glucose infused over 24 hours without any side-effects. However, caution is advised if your patient has any of the following characteristics: is very young or very old, has signs of septicaemia, is severely malnourished, is taking steroids, or is a diabetic. Due to the high content of glucose as a calorie source in PN, careful monitoring of glucose is essential.

Intolerance of glucose is signalled by the presence of glucose in the urine (glycosuria), which may lead to an increase in diuresis and result in dehydration of the patient. If untreated, the patient may show an abnormally high level of glucose in the blood (hyperglycaemia), which could lead to acidosis and potential death. It is therefore important that this problem is recognised early and treated appropriately. Urinalysis should be performed on a daily basis for those patients who appear to have stable conditions and have no history of glucose intolerance. However, patients who have any of the previous characteristics will require more careful monitoring. If glucose is present in the urine, then a formal blood sugar level test will be required, and the patient should be observed for signs of hyperglycaemia, i.e. dehydration, excessive urinary output, headache and confusion. If hyperglycaemia is confirmed after medical assessment, the patient may require intravenous fluid replacement, and either subcutaneous or intravenous insulin, depending on the severity of the condition and local medical policies.

If glycosuria occurs in a patient who has had no previous problems with glucose tolerance, then it is also important to check the following (Grant 1992):

- *The rate of the infusion.* A rapid increase in rate may be due to incorrect setting of the infusion pump; a deliberate increase in rate because the infusion was behind schedule; or it may be that no infusion pump was used, and the gravity drip, which has fewer safeguards, infuses too quickly. A positive urinalysis for glucose in these cases will indicate that the infusion will need to be slowed, and the patient observed for hyperglycaemia.

• *Concomitant medications*. Other drugs that the patient is receiving at the same time as the PN infusion may interfere with glucose metabolism. Steroid treatment, which has been mentioned previously, can initiate glyconeogenesis, leading to hyperglycaemia. Some diuretics can deplete potassium levels, resulting in a higher glucose level, and phenytoin in high doses leads to slower insulin secretion in the body.

• *Temperature*. The stress response by the human body to sepsis can lead to glucose being present in the urine up to 12 h prior to there being any clinical signs.

• *Potassium blood levels*. A low blood potassium level has been shown in many studies to result in glucose intolerance and glycosuria. The mechanism of why this occurs is complex, and is determined by many variables.

It is also important to consider the effect of a strong glucose infusion on the respiratory system. An increased level of carbohydrate metabolism, caused by the infusion of glucose, leads to an increased production of carbon dioxide. Normally, an adult will compensate adequately for this, and research indicates that it may require an excessive rise in an individual's carbohydrate intake to produce this effect. However, it can cause problems with patients who are requiring assisted ventilation, or those who have respiratory disease.

An abnormally low blood glucose level (hypoglycaemia) is usually the result of the parenteral infusion being abruptly stopped. In this case the patient may have symptoms of clammy skin, thirst, dizziness, headaches and an increased pulse rate. He will therefore require oral or intravenous carbohydrate to raise his blood glucose level to normal. It is therefore suggested that the patient, where possible, be slowly weaned from the PN, and that the cessation of the infusion at night be avoided wherever possible. This is covered in more detail in Chapter 8.

Hypophosphataemia

Depleted levels of phosphate may be due to a variety of disorders from malabsorption syndromes to alcoholism. Administration of PN solutions that do not contain phosphate supplements can lead to depleted levels of phosphate. Typically patients with low phosphate levels show symptoms of muscle weakness, particularly of the jaw and neck, and may show paraesthesia of their extremities. Treatment is by phosphate supplementation, and avoidance of hypophosphataemia by correct administration through PN infusions. It is important to note also that there is an increase in renal excretion of phosphate in patients who have hypokalaemia, hypomagnesaemia, diabetes mellitus and during steroid and diuretic treatment. These patients may require the parenteral infusion to be compensated, if any of these problems occur.

Hypomagnesaemia

Magnesium is an important ion due to its role in the activation of enzymes that are essential to cell metabolism (Grant 1992). A low magnesium level is typically seen in the patients who have gastrointestinal disorders, resulting in the patient experiencing muscle weakness, tremors, spasticity and ataxia. The patient may also display mood disturbances ranging from depression and irritability to apathy and psychotic behaviour. Nausea and vomiting is also another side-effect, and severe deficiencies can lead to convulsions. Since many of these symptoms are similar to those of hypocalcaemia, it is important that the problem is confirmed through biochemical analysis of a blood sample. Magnesium levels will require maintenance throughout the PN infusion period, and a low magnesium level will need to be corrected by intravenous infusion.

Hypermagnesaemia

This problem usually occurs in patients with renal failure, and can lead to the patients experiencing hypotension, nausea and vomiting, and in extreme cases can result in cardiac arrest. Serum magnesium analysis will be required at regular intervals, so that an appropriate amount of magnesium can be supplemented to the parenteral solution. In cases of extremely high levels of magnesium, renal dialysis is indicated.

Lipid metabolism complications

Infusion of lipid solutions can cause the following problems.

High serum triglyceride levels. A high serum triglyceride (also called triacylglycerol) level after the infusion of lipid emulsions has been shown in some studies to be associated with the abnormal functioning of the liver, kidneys and pancreas, and has also been linked to blood coagulation irregularities and immune disorders. This high level is usually caused by the rapid infusion of the lipid substance; therefore, as previously mentioned, it is important that the infusion is carefully monitored and regulated, so that the problem can be avoided.

Essential fatty acid deficiency. Fatty acids play an important role within the body for maintaining membrane structure and integrity. If a patient is deficient in these essential fatty acids, then he will experience symptoms of dryness, thickening, and scaling of the skin. This side-effect will initially become apparent on the face, skinfolds and extremities, and will then gradually spread to the rest of the body. The patient's hair will become more coarse and alopecia may occur. Poor wound healing will also be a problem, and this will be further complicated by anaemia and thrombocytopenia. Many of these side-effects have been noted in patients who have not had lipid included in their PN; it is therefore important that this potential problem is addressed at the time of prescribing the PN infusion. Administration of lipids, and in particular linolenic acid, will correct the deficiency symptoms within 2–3 weeks.

Hyperammonaemia

A high blood ammonia level is commonly seen in children receiving PN. The reduction in cases of hyperammonaemia in adults is thought to be due to the introduction of crystalline amino acid formulations for use in PN solutions. These crystalline amino acid preparations contain no ammonia, in contrast to the previous hydrolysate amino acid solutions, which contained ammonia. The majority of adults who do experience high levels of ammonia frequently exhibit a degree of liver disease; however, there are usually no clinical signs of the problem. Ammonia in the body is converted to urea by a mechanism called the Krebs cycle. Arginine, an amino acid, plays an important part within the cycle in assisting in the conversion of ammonia to urea, and a deficiency of arginine may lead to hyperammonaemia. Since hyperammonaemia is reported most commonly in paediatric and neonate patients, formulations of PN will usually contain a higher amount of arginine.

A child suffering from hyperammonaemia will exhibit signs of decreased responsiveness, followed by twitching which can lead to seizures and coma.

Trace element abnormalities

Zinc. Zinc is an important element required for enzyme metabolism and DNA synthesis. Deficiencies can lead to abnormal taste and smell, growth retardation, changes in mood, poor wound healing, poor white cell function, alopecia, rashes and diarrhoea. If PN is administered without zinc supplements, then it is likely that these complications will occur after 2 weeks.

Copper. Copper is an important element required for enzyme action. A low level of copper in an adult may result in anaemia and neutropenia. In children osteoporosis has been reported. In general, a deficiency is only seen in patients who are requiring long-term PN and have not received adequate supplements. However, it must be noted that requirements for copper may increase if a patient is experiencing severe diarrhoea.

Hepatic complications

In the past, a rise in the level of serum liver enzymes was a common occurrence in patients receiving PN. Today, some patients may still have a rise in their levels after about 10–14 days after the commencement of the infusion, but the frequency of this complication is gradually declining. The mechanism for this occurrence is still not clear, but it is thought that previous policies of rapidly infusing high dextrose solutions may have played some part in this process. In the past 10 years the introduction of lipid infusions as an alternative energy source to glucose infusions has supported this theory, since more recent studies have indicated lower rises in serum liver enzyme levels.

Fatty infiltration of the liver, or steatosis, is also a complication thought to be a result of high dextrose infusions, and is characterised by a rise in the patient's liver function tests (LFTs). This rise is commonly seen after 5 days of starting the PN infusion and the problem usually resolves quickly after the infusion is stopped.

Gall bladder problems and cholestasis are also potential problems associated with long-term PN. Lack of stimulation of the bile duct causes limited emptying of the gall bladder and leads to the formation of sludge and possibly gallstones. In some cases acute cholecystitis can occur, even if there are no gallstones present. These problems usually resolve once normal feeding has been established.

Hypoalbuminaemia

Albumin plays an important role in the body for the distribution and transportation of many substances including blood and fatty acids. A low albumin level is associated with those who are severely malnourished, have cancer, have liver cirrhosis, or are stressed due to infection, trauma, surgery or burns. This results in lower resistance to infection, poor wound healing and impaired absorption of fluid and electrolytes from the gut. However, the role of albumin supplementation is not clear. Some studies indicate that adding albumin to parenteral nutrition solutions improves a patient's morbidity, whereas other studies explain that this approach is fraught with problems. One of these problems is the increased rate of bacterial and fungal growth in PN solution containing albumin. Another problem points to the association of an increase in occluded line filters due to strong albumin concentrations. In general it is suggested that albumin should be infused separately to the PN solution, and further analysis is required to clarify the evidence of whether albumin supplementation improves clinical outcome (Grant 1992).

Fluid and electrolyte complications

Patients receiving PN will require the same careful monitoring and evaluation of fluid balance as any patient receiving intravenous fluid therapy. Since PN is not an emergency procedure, attention should be paid to correcting any electrolyte imbalance prior to commencement of the treatment. The patient's current cardiac and renal functions are particularly important since abnormalities of these systems may predispose the patient to fluid retention and overload. It is also important to consider other factors such as potential fluid loss from stomas, fistulae or diarrhoea, since this will impact on the amount and type of replacement fluid required. If the patient is dehydrated he may well become thirsty and there will be a reduction in the amount of urine passed. The patient will also have an elevated level of serum sodium, and if fluid replacement is not performed, then stupor, coma and death may ensue. If the patient is over hydrated he will pass urine more frequently and his body weight will increase. A reduction in the patient's oral fluid intake or the careful use of diuretic medications may therefore be appropriate.

The infusion of glucose solutions can also increase the insulin demand by the body, and result in the redistribution of potassium into the cells. This may be indicated by a fall in the level of serum potassium shown through biochemical analysis. Close monitoring of this level, and subsequent changes to the PN infusion solution, may be required.

Metabolic bone disease

Metabolic bone disease is characterised by pathological fractures or leg and back pain. This may be a consequence of long-term PN therapy, but the mechanism for this disease progression is not fully known; however, the evidence appears to point towards the involvement of vitamin D. Stopping the administration of vitamin D, or discontinuing the PN infusion, leads to a resolution of the symptoms, but remineralisation of the bone may take many months, if not years.

CONCLUSION

This chapter has examined closely complications associated with the use of PN. The first section analysed the range of problems related to long-term indwelling cvcs. It was shown that, whatever product was used to assist in the management of these problems, it was vital for the professional to establish an evidence-based protocol, and to review this protocol on a regular basis.

The next section of the chapter discussed mechanical complications relating to the infusion of the PN. Finally, metabolic complications arising as a result of the administration of PN were examined in some detail. These were related not only to the systemic effects, but also most importantly to the clinical signs that a patient may experience.

REFERENCES

Brandt B, De Palma J, Irwin M, Shogan J, Lucke JF 1996 Comparison of central venous catheter dressings in bone marrow transplant recipients. Oncology Nursing Forum 23(5):829–836

Cunha BA 1995 Diagnosis and prevention of intravenous central line-associated infections. Heart and Lung 24(4):261–262

Grant JP 1992 Septic and metabolic complications: recognition and management. In: Grant JP (ed) Handbook of total parenteral nutrition, 2nd edn. WB Saunders, Philadelphia

Haire WD, Lieberman RP, Lund GB, Edney J, Wieczorek BM 1990 Obstructed central venous catheters: restoring function with a 12 hour infusion of Urokinase. Cancer 66:2279–2285

Hamilton H 1993 Care improves whilst costs reduce. Professional Nurse 8(9):592–596

Hoffmann KK, Weber DJ, Samsa GP 1992 Transparent polyurethane film as an intravenous catheter dressing. Journal of the American Medical Association 267:2072–2076

Kelly C, Dimenko L, McGregor SE, McHutchion ME 1992 A change in flushing protocols of central venous catheters. Oncology Nursing Forum 19(4):599–605

Lawson ML, Kavanagh T, McCredie K, Marts K, Barbour N, Chandler W 1986 Comparison of transparent dressings to paper tape dressing over central venous catheter sites. National Intravenous Therapy Association 9(1):40–43

Maki DG 1991 Infection caused by intravascular devices: pathogenesis, strategies for prevention. In: Maki DG (ed) Improving catheter site care. Royal Society of Medicine Services Ltd, London

Maki DG, McCormack KN 1987 Defatting catheter insertion sites in total parenteral nutrition is of no value as an infection control measure. American Journal of Medicine 83:833–840

Maki DG, Ringer M, Alvarado CJ 1991 Prospective randomised trial of povidone iodine, alcohol and chlorhexidine for prevention of infection associated with central venous and arterial catheters. Lancet 338:339–343

Perry C, Leaper D 1994 Care of central venous line exit sites. Journal of Wound Care. 3(6):279–282

Raad II, Luna M, Khahl SAM, Costerton JW, Lam C, Bodey GP 1994 The relationship between thrombotic and infectious complications of central venous catheters. Journal of the American Medical Association 271(13):1014–1016

Tolar B, Gould JR 1996 The timing and sequence of multiple device-related complications in patients with long term indwelling Groshong catheters. Cancer 78(6):1308–1313

10

Home parenteral nutrition

Sally Magnay

Introduction
Coming to terms with HPN
Education of patients/carers prior to
    discharge on HPN
Training programme

Equipment required for HPN
Home assessment
Discharge
Monitoring and complications
Conclusion

INTRODUCTION

Home-administered nutritional support is an expanding aspect of healthcare. Advances in technology now ensure safe and effective administration of both parenteral and enteral nutrition within the home. Home parenteral nutrition (HPN) has been available in the UK since the late 1970s and the ability to treat established intestinal failure with prolonged parenteral nutrition (PN) is well established (Jeejeeboy 1983). In the past PN was usually only considered appropriate for the long-term patient with intestinal failure. However, due to the pressure on acute hospital beds, the concept of HPN for a period of weeks or months is not uncommon. As a result of empirical knowledge and more widespread expertise in centres caring for patients receiving HPN, a greater number of people with long-term intestinal failure now have greater life expectancies and also enjoy a relatively full life with minimal complications.

The indication for HPN is permanent intestinal failure, and in the UK the most frequent indication is short bowel syndrome, often related to Crohn's disease. Other indications may include radiation enteritis secondary to treatment for cancer. In the USA HPN is often utilised in patients with inoperable malignancies, essentially improving the quality of life, but this is not generally advocated in the UK.

COMING TO TERMS WITH HPN

Patients requiring HPN usually have an underlying disease process that may already be causing them psychological stress. When faced with the prospect of another alteration to their lives, they understandably feel overwhelmed.

In order for the multidisciplinary team to enable the patient to cope and accept HPN, members may need to be aware of the natural and common reactions that may manifest in a patient's attitudes and behaviour. Feelings of resentment and fear may occur. These are normal reactions and should be encouraged to be expressed freely within a supportive, non-judgemental framework. Strong communication links within the team encourage members to be aware of the appropriate information related to the patient's psychological state and promote good collaborative practice.

A patient with long-term or permanent loss of body functions necessitating artificial nutritional support at home requires additional support; the organisation and provision of the practicalities to facilitate successful administration of PN in the home is only a very small part of the care required. Psychological adaptation is successfully achieved only after the process of acceptance has truly occurred. The ability to cope with trauma and hardship varies considerably between individuals. The implications to some people's psychological well being after the loss of a major body function will be greater than to others.

The nutrition nurse specialist is perhaps the most appropriate person to take time to discuss and familiarise herself with the patient, promoting a relationship that encourages honest and free expression. It is the basis of this relationship that will enable the nurse to communicate effectively to other members of the team the patient's anxieties and needs.

The nurse usually provides a safe and trusting environment for the patient, motivating them to communicate their anxieties and fears. The nurse can coordinate and liaise with peripheral disciplines and agencies that may be required in order to facilitate 'complete' holistic care. For example, it may be felt by the team that the patient would benefit from a psychological assessment to promote a greater understanding of their disease process and the implications to their lifestyle. As a result, the appropriate treatment and support can be arranged by the team accordingly.

The nurse will also be aware of the financial implications that HPN may have on the patient and the family. A benefits expert from Social Services can assist with advice and support, additionally addressing rehousing concerns or assisting in the completion of necessary form filling.

A patient who is unable to progress through the grief stage of loss and feels constantly regretful for her past way of life may find it difficult to move forward and construct new ways of living and being. Depression is not uncommon when the patient becomes aware of the effect that artificial nutritional support, with all its implications, will have on family life and hobbies. Intimate sexual relations are frequently affected by anxiety and inhibition surrounding the presence of an exiting central catheter on the chest wall. Frustration and resentment are often experienced, particularly by the young person, who understandably feels distressed by the restrictions to his or her lifestyle that are involved, to a greater or lesser extent, by receiving HPN.

Some patients are unable to express openly and directly their anger and frustration at what fate has dealt them, and instead direct it to complaints regarding the PN administration system or members of the team caring for them. In assessing any communication with these patients it is very important to possess an objective mind, and keep things in perspective.

A patient feels reassured and secure if she believes she has an empathetic, compassionate advocate in the nurse responsible for her HPN, who is prepared throughout her admission, training process and on discharge to accompany her emotionally, and support and provide expert professional, sympathetic care.

Realistic, compassionate responses by the NST to a patient's emotional feelings are vital and should continue during the often protracted period of time that HPN may be necessary. Once the decision has been made to discharge a patient home on HPN, the type of venous access device must be determined. This is usually a tunnelled central venous catheter or a subcutaneous port, both of which are described in detail in Chapter 4.

EDUCATION OF PATIENTS/CARERS PRIOR TO DISCHARGE ON HPN

The training process of a patient or their carer in the techniques required for safe delivery of PN requires careful planning and appropriate guidance and supervision. The British Association for Parenteral and Enteral Nutrition (BAPEN 1995) has produced a booklet outlining *Learning Goals* and a standard for discharge that should be achieved 24 h prior to discharge. The BAPEN guidelines provide specific, clear and measurable objectives for the patient and her carers (see Table 10.1). Comprehensive, invaluable information regarding all aspects relating to HPN are covered within this publication.

The establishment of a good learning environment plus teacher/learner relationship is of fundamental importance. Effectively assessing the level of the patient/carer's understanding regarding gastrointestinal function, PN, how it is delivered to the body and how it is absorbed will provide the nurse with a clear base to work from.

Patient assessment and learning checks are very important and may reveal that many patients have little knowledge of the workings of their bodies, frequently expressing gross misinterpretations.

Prior to active training, the nutrition support team (NST) need to collaborate and decide upon the patient's suitability for training, e.g.:

- If recovering postoperatively, is the patient physically strong enough to perform the procedures?
- If malnourished, the patient may have poor concentration span, be apathetic and listless.
- Is the patient psychologically prepared to undertake the training to accomplishment process as a result of their inability to accept the

Table 10.1 BAPEN guidelines for preparing the patient for HPN (BAPEN 1995)

Structure	Process	Outcome
There will be a training programme for healthcare professionals involved in the care of patients receiving home intravenous nutrition.	Discharge planning will be performed only by professionals who have the necessary experience or who have undertaken a course of training in the topic.	The patient has confidence in the hospital team planning his/her discharge.
There will be a model of care for patients needing home intravenous nutrition.	All members of the multidisciplinary team will be involved in writing the 'mission statement' on which the model is based.	The patient will know the beliefs, aims and objectives of the HPN Care Team.
There will be a relaxed, quiet area suitable for private discussion.	There will be a caring and compassionate atmosphere with adequate time for discussion.	The patient will feel able to express his/her fears and expectations.
The discharge planning documentation will include sections on domestic, family and social circumstances.	The nutrition team will evaluate with the patient and family how the HPN will alter his/her way of life.	The patient will believe that the feeding system can be integrated into an acceptable way of life.
There will be written patient/carer learning goals for HPN.	A designated nurse will be responsible for teaching the patient according to his/her capacity for learning.	The patient/carer will be able to demonstrate the necessary skills and achieve all the individual learning goals.
There will be an instruction manual for home intravenous nutrition.	Information and procedures will be regularly updated in order to reflect developments and innovations in venous access, nutrient solutions and delivery systems.	The patient will perform therapy based on current practice.
A relative, friend or appropriate healthcare professional will be able to deliver therapy if the patient is unable to do so (e.g. parent or guardian of a child).	The healthcare professional will help the patient to identify the most appropriate carer. The district nurse will be given the opportunity to visit the patient in hospital and observe therapy before the patient is discharged.	The patient has confidence that safe care will be available at home.
Venous access will be achieved by a central venous catheter suitable for long-term use.	The patient, nurse and doctor will choose the most appropriate catheter and access site.	The patient will use a central venous catheter that is acceptable and accessible.
There will be written procedures for the management of central venous catheters.	The nurse will adapt the procedures according to the patient's physical skills and domestic circumstances.	The patient's daily life will not be restricted by prolonged inappropriate procedures.
Written information describing HPN will be available for the GP.	The hospital teams will provide the GP with the information before the patient is discharged, together with the	The patient will have confidence in his/her GP's knowledge of HPN.

Table 10.1   (*contd*)

Structure	Process	Outcome
	discharge date, and on-call telephone numbers.	
There will be a written prescription for the nutrition solutions (and other prescribable items).	The patient's GP will be contacted and advised on how to prescribe the feed.	The patient will have the feeding solution available at home on the day of discharge.
There will be a list of the required equipment, e.g. refrigerator, infusion pump, syringes, sterile gloves, telephone.	Before discharge, the patient's home health authority will be provided with the list and asked to arrange supply by making local arrangements or establishing a contract with a commercial supplier.	The patient will have all the necessary supplies at home on the day of discharge.
There will be an on-call system for providing expert advice to the patient by telephone day and night.	The nurse will explain the system to the patient and identify the professions involved.	The patient/carer will know the names and telephone numbers to contact in case of an emergency by day or night.
Information will be available describing how the nutrient solutions and supplies will be provided following discharge.	The nurse will explain the chosen supply system and discuss storage depending on the patient's home circumstances.	The patient will know how to obtain supplies, store them and dispose of unwanted material.
There will be a post-discharge discharge monitoring protocol, established by the nutrition team.	Monitoring will be supervised by the nutrition team.	The patient will know the date of the first outpatient visit and what monitoring will be performed.

necessary treatment? The patient may be in denial, angry or resentful that artificial nutrition has become a necessity.

• In relation to the severity of their condition – is it unlikely that they will ever be appropriate for HPN training?

• Manual dexterity impairment caused by rheumatoid arthritis or scleroderma for example, may mean that the patient is unable to perform technical procedures.

If the reason for a delay in commencement of training is related to insufficient postoperative recovery or undernourished state, a delay will hopefully be short. However, if, following assessment, it is decided that the patient is unlikely to safely undergo training, a carer needs to be identified. Each patient has a unique set of circumstances and lifestyle and these will need to be considered carefully by the patient, carer and nurse. A district nursing team providing comprehensive cover can successfully deliver the required care if the patient resides in an area where community services are not too overutilised. Unfortunately, the feasibility of district nurse cover cannot always be assumed, and discussion with the patient, relatives and friends is therefore required to investigate the possibility of a suitable, willing carer. This may be a partner or, in the case of a patient living alone, a small group of people.

BAPEN recommends that: 'The health care professional helps the patient to identify the most appropriate carer. District nurses should be provided with the opportunity to visit the patient in hospital and observe therapy prior to discharge' (BAPEN 1995).

Each patient/carer training process is to an extent uniquely created and adapted for that person, taking into consideration the knowledge and understanding the nurse has about them. However, the basic format of learning, guidance and supervision leading to independence will be the same for everyone. The time span for accomplishment of independence varies according to individual abilities, but an estimate is between 2 and 3 weeks.

TRAINING PROGRAMME

The first stage of the training programme consists of theoretical sessions taking place in a quiet, uninterrupted, comfortable environment. Useful literature resources include patient information booklets produced by the hospital or literature available from the patients' association – Patients on Intravenous and Nasogastric Nutrition Therapy (PINNT). These are helpful as they have been carefully written to meet the requirements of the non-medical person.

In the preliminary theoretical sessions the principles of normal intestinal function and how these have changed due to intestinal failure should be covered. Once the concept of PN is understood – what it is, where it is delivered and what happens when it enters the body – discussion can progress to the principles of asepsis. The importance of asepsis throughout training will be strongly emphasised. The patient/carer needs to understand clearly the methods used to ensure strict asepsis and the consequences if these principles are not adhered to.

The procedures (according to hospital/BAPEN protocol) involved in administering PN and caring for the venous access device are performed initially by the nurse. It is preferable that the training is undertaken by a key person in order to provide continuity and standardisation of care. The patient/carer is encouraged to observe closely and ask questions during these procedures. The nurse should explain the rationale behind the methods used and answer any questions as they arise.

In the early stages, providing the patient/carer with some of the equipment to familiarise themselves with, and then practise using, breaks down some of the barriers and anxieties that may have developed. Donning a pair of sterile gloves in an aseptic fashion and drawing up a syringe of water requires a high degree of psychomotor skill. Repetition in a relaxed, non-threatening practice setting enables the operator to develop confidence and competence. Aids for the accomplishment of these skills such as a doll with a venous access device strapped to the chest wall, or simply a piece of hardboard with a chest depicted and access device deposited on it, may be deployed in order for the patient/carer to practise safely procedures related to catheter management.

It is important that the teaching sessions are conducted with the minimum of stress in order to facilitate the most conducive learning environment, and appropriately staged according to the individual's needs. The nurse aids the process by empathetic and observant verbal and non-verbal communication, and by objectively meeting the interpretation of these signs gently and appropriately.

Once the patient/carer in combination with the nurse feels ready to perform the actual procedures, careful attention to timing and setting are important. At the bedside with the curtains drawn, adequate lighting, sufficient space, and at a time when you are unlikely to be disturbed by medical rounds, investigations or visitors, provides the ideal setting. Support and guidance by the nurse during the practice of the psychomotor skills can be given in a respectful, non-threatening way. Providing positive feedback when appropriate aids in building up the patient's self-confidence.

The patient/carer is educated about the pump, which will deliver the PN, how it works, what to do when it alarms, how to care for it and what to do if it fails. A clear understanding about the central venous catheter (cvc), the position within the body and what care this requires is essential for the HPN patient. The patient/carer should be encouraged to view the catheter as a precious commodity, as it is hoped that it will be reliable and last for a long period of time. Many HPN patients have successfully retained the same cvc in excess of 6 years, when it eventually wore out! Again, local policy dictates the type of catheter, the number of lumens, and which clamping devices are applied.

Access devices can be characterised by the number and size of the catheter lumen and by whether an external connector or implantable port terminates the catheter. Most HPN patients have an external segment catheter, e.g. a Broviac or Hickman type device. Many patients find this type of catheter acceptable; however, in order to ensure that a patient's preferences are fully taken into consideration, the various access devices should be explained carefully to her at an early stage in her training.

The Hickman or Broviac style catheter, when managed correctly, is a satisfactory device with which to provide long-term PN. However, there are disadvantages to the HPN patient in terms of certain specific social aspects, e.g. body image and the freedom to shower or swim without restrictions. The use of implantable ports provides an alternative and those patients who have experienced external catheters state that a port imposes fewer restrictions in the choice of clothes and facilitates sporting activities, particularly those involving water. Additionally, the patient is less anxious when involved in sexual activity and generally lifestyle is less impeded by the presence of an external access device. The repeated needle sticks required to access the port may be intolerable or undesirable for many patients, particularly those requiring nightly PN.

While peripherally inserted central catheters (PICCs) are gaining in popularity in many centres for the short- to medium-term delivery of PN, they have not yet been used for prolonged periods for the administration of PN. The absence of a Dacron cuff and the position in the antecubital fossa means that their immobility cannot be guaranteed.

Guidelines on the appropriate response to a suspected infection of a cvc need to be given verbally and in written form. The patient should be provided with a 24 h contact telephone number for advice from a member of the NST who can then, if necessary, arrange emergency admission. The patient's GP should also be provided with appropriate emergency contact numbers and made fully conversant with the appropriate actions in the event of a suspected infection associated with the PN catheter.

Identification of complications in the verbal and written form must be provided with clear instructions regarding what to do in the event of an emergency.

Complications may include:

- catheter-related sepsis
- catheter occlusion
- venous thrombosis
- catheter fracture
- hypo/hyperglycaemia.

The importance of monitoring the cvc used for PN must be covered prior to the patient's discharge.

During training, the patient may be encouraged to take responsibility for self-monitoring in preparation for discharge. This may include monitoring fluid balance, daily weights, and urinalysis for the detection of glycosuria, in addition to monitoring the cvc. As a patient/carer becomes increasingly confident and competent in the performance of the procedures, independence should be encouraged. However, support and guidance should still be readily available.

Pre-discharge training will also include knowledge about appropriate storage of PN, guidelines regarding the checking of the PN prior to use, and how the PN will be delivered to the patient's home, when and by whom. A home monitoring protocol will have been established by the NST and should accompany the patient on discharge.

EQUIPMENT REQUIRED FOR HPN

Prior to a home assessment, the nurse should consider the type and quantity of equipment the patient will require at discharge. The nurse responsible for the patient's safe and effective discharge needs to bear in mind that, first and foremost, this is the patient's home – PN should be incorporated into the patient's life and not dominate it. Therefore, the home should not adopt the look of a mini hospital or clinic. With care and creativity the nurse can ensure that the patient is provided with equipment that is discreet and easily managed.

Dressing trolley

Folding varieties are available and can be stored when not in use. Some patients may find a stainless steel or plastic tray will provide a clean surface on which to perform sterile procedures. This is often advisable if the patient is travelling or away from her normal environment. The tray should be cleaned in the same way as a dressing trolley.

Drip stand

One standard hospital-type drip stand is recommended for the commencement of PN. However, smaller designs are also available, making movement over carpet much easier. Modern designs can be folded, making them more discreet and allowing ease of travel, etc.

Electronic pump

The majority of HPN patients are supplied with a pump that attaches to a drip stand. However, with modern technology lighter, more sophisticated pumps are now available to give HPN patients more freedom of mobility.

Several versions of portable pumps are available and are either completely operator programmable or preprogrammed using a bar code generated by the NST. Portable pumps are placed within a backpack containing the PN bag. This allows the patient to enjoy considerable freedom and provides greater flexibility with daily living activities within the home and work environment. This type of pump is of particular benefit to those patients requiring long infusion times owing to large fluid requirements. The disadvantage to the provision of such pumps is cost. However, every effort should be made by the nurse to state a strong case to managers for patients, particularly those requiring permanent PN, to enjoy a quality of life that technology of this type can provide.

Parenteral nutrition should always be administered via a pump with clear, user-friendly controls, indicators and displays. The pump should have an alarm system and be accompanied by sound and safe explanations of how to deal with problems as they occur. Infusion pumps must be regularly serviced and in the event of a breakdown a system must be in place where a prompt replacement of the pump is assured.

Refrigerator

A refrigerator of sufficient size, maintained at a constant temperature of 4°C, and designated exclusively for the storage of PN is required. This should be large enough to enable single storage of PN bags and avoid bags being piled on top of one another.

Under the auspices of BAPEN a multidisciplinary group has been set up to consider equipment necessary for the patient requiring PN. This group is called LITRE – Looking Into the Requirements for Equipment. The aim of this group is to respond to patients/carers concerned about equipment related to the infusion of PN and to work closely with industry in order that appropriate technological advances can be made in future designs of this equipment.

HOME ASSESSMENT

Prior to discharge, a home visit by the nurse should take place to ensure that home circumstances are suitable for this type of community therapy. At a suitable time, a home visit and assessment should be arranged. The nurse needs to ascertain the suitability of the home environment for HPN and, if necessary, organise and coordinate any work that may be required to make sure the home circumstances are suitable for the delivery of intravenous nutrition. Structural alterations may be necessary for some patients who, following prolonged periods in hospital, may be unable to climb stairs, or who may require dedicated washbasin facilities. These alterations should be completed prior to the patient's discharge.

Considerations that the nurse will be required to make should include:

- sufficient, safe and accessible power points
- adequate space for safe storage of sterile equipment in a clean, dry area
- space for designated PN fridge
- dedicated suite for handwashing close to the area where sterile procedures are to be performed.

Attention is paid to the area within the patient's home where procedures for setting up the PN infusion and discontinuing it are going to be performed. Ideally a designated clean room close to a sink, on the same floor where the patient will retire to bed, is required. The nurse will pay attention to the type of floor coverings, which may highlight difficulties when the patient attempts to push a drip stand over a carpeted area.

Recommending the placement of a plastic carpet protector may be an option to facilitate the mobility of the drip stand.

Clearly, pets should be kept away from stored equipment and during sterile procedures. However, providing they are not likely to cause harm to the patient and sterile equipment, it is unnecessary for pets to be banned.

The nurse performing the home assessment is responsible for providing advice regarding equipment storage, the type of containers to be used, and how and where they are placed. Direction on the most appropriate area for procedures and on which floor of the house/flat will also be of use to the patient. Adaptations such as shelves and the use of plastic stacking storage containers facilitate compact storage of large amounts of ancillaries. The position of power points requires careful consideration and the addition of extra power points is often required.

There will be occasions where, on assessment, the home environment is found to be unsuitable, owing to various factors. These may include cramped conditions, limited storage space, unhygienic environment, or unsatisfactory sanitary conditions. If the patient is a council tenant an appeal for re-housing or an extension to the existing property may be required. However, on most occasions discussion, reorganisation and a little creativity usually surmount most problems.

DISCHARGE

Many hospitals make use of commercial companies for the delivery of ancillary goods and PN directly to the patient's home. These companies undertake to provide a quality service to the patient and maintain close liaison with the patient and NST attached to the referring hospital.

It is routine for the commercial company to provide the patient with all the equipment that is necessary to administer PN. As detailed above, the equipment will include a drip stand, folding dressing trolley and a refrigerator to be used specifically and exclusively for PN. This refrigerator will be kept at a temperature of 4°C. The selected commercial company will undertake to communicate on a regular basis directly with the patient/carer regarding stock levels, delivery dates and times. In addition, many companies will also deliver PN to alternative addresses or holiday venues, throughout the world if necessary.

Prior to discharging a patient requiring HPN, permission must be sought from the Medical Advisor for the health authority concerned. The authority must provide written confirmation for acceptance of the costs for the patient on an ongoing basis (Department of Health EL (95) Purchasing of High Tech Healthcare for Patients in the Community). Some health authorities may have contracts with specific home care suppliers, while others may expect the nurse responsible for the patient's discharge to recommend a suitable company. If this is the case, then it is advisable to obtain a variety of quotes for the various suppliers as, depending on the nutritional requirements of the patient, prices can vary enormously.

To aid in the selection of a company, BAPEN provide a standard for the supply of PN and equipment in their publication: *Home Parenteral Nutrition – Quality Criteria for Clinical Services and the Supply of Nutritional Fluids and Equipment* (BAPEN 1995b). Any healthcare company that is used will be required to meet the criteria stated in this document.

On the day of discharge it is often usual for the nurse to accompany the patient home, or at least attend the following day to ensure all the equipment, PN and sterile goods are in place. In addition the nurse will provide the reassurance and support necessary for the performance of procedures in a new environment. The patient/carer will have instruction manuals or crib cards, often individually devised during the training period to hand and will be able to contact the nurse by phone if anxieties arise.

Recommendations of BAPEN state that on discharge the patient/carer will be able to:

- change the dressing covering the cvc in an aseptic way
- connect the PN infusion to the catheter aseptically
- program the infusion pump safely
- disconnect the infusion and flush the cvc
- recognise thrombosis and catheter occlusion
- contact the appropriate healthcare professional when necessary.

Written information describing HPN will be provided to the GP and district nursing team prior to the patient's discharge. The GP and district nurses should be informed in advance of the patient's discharge date, on-call telephone numbers and the date of the first outpatients appointment. The following information should be supplied:

- a discharge letter outlining the continuing treatment programme and outpatient appointment date;
- background information of HPN;
- advice regarding common complications of PN and guidance on what emergency action to be taken;
- guidance on the contribution and responsibilities of the GP, local hospital and NST;
- emergency protocols should complications occur;
- contact telephone number of the nurse member of the NST.

MONITORING AND COMPLICATIONS

A designated form is useful for this purpose and should contain a record of the patient's current weight, body mass index (BMI) and the mid arm muscle circumference. These records will provide a baseline measurement for future monitoring. During hospitalisation laboratory measurements for haematology and biochemistry, liver function, zinc and magnesium will have been assessed several times a week. In addition, strict fluid balance, daily weight, 4-hourly temperature, pulse and respiration and twice daily urinalysis will have been monitored. On discharge the same level of monitoring is not necessary.

In the early days of PN fluid and electrolyte abnormalities are common and hyperglycaemia is a frequent occurrence, particularly in relation to cyclic infusions of PN. These teething problems will have been addressed prior to discharge, resulting in the maximum stability of the patient at discharge. However, it should be stressed to the patient/carer that manipulation of the administration time of PN is hazardous. Any alteration to the infusion time should be discussed with the NST.

Fluid and volume intolerance may affect infusion time, creating difficulties for the patient wishing to attend work, etc. The patient should be alerted to potential symptoms such as nocturnal dyspnoea, ankle oedema or sudden swings in weight pattern and the significance of these explained.

The most common and serious complication associated with HPN is related neither to the nutritional content nor the metabolic response to this, but rather to the catheter. Catheter-related sepsis is usually caused by *Staphylococcus aureus* or *S. epidermidis*, skin-related organisms that often occur due to poor aseptic technique or a relaxed approach to catheter care. It is therefore very important that the patient appreciates the need for fastidious monitoring and detailed technique in the maintenance of the PN, whilst enjoying the pleasure of returning home to family and friends.

The HPN patient will initially require weekly biochemical assessment to ensure that stability is maintained. Haematological assessment may also be performed on a weekly basis initially. Once full stability is reached, the NST and clinician may feel that all metabolic investigations can be performed fortnightly, or even monthly. Three-monthly micronutrient screening and vitamin and trace element analysis are advisable on the severely depleted patient, and for those patients who are almost entirely dependent on intravenous nutrition, ensuring that the levels of vitamins, trace elements and micronutrients added to the PN are meeting the individual patients' requirements. Clinical, laboratory and nutritional monitoring takes place on attendance at the nutrition outpatients appointment, alongside quality of life assessment and PN catheter performance.

This regular assessment by the NST is of particular importance when considering growth and development of children or adolescents receiving PN.

CONCLUSION

As the move toward reduced length of hospital stay and community-based therapy continues, the use of HPN will undoubtedly increase. Monitoring and evaluation of the success of such patients is an essential role of the NST and will aid in ensuring that future patients will benefit from experiences gained in this intensive and costly method of nutrition.

HPN can be a very successful therapy, but it can also place exceptional strain on family relationships. A skilled nurse in this field can provide invaluable support to this group of patients and their families, encouraging independence, designing coping strategies in a follow-up programme and generally acting as their confidante.

Patient support groups are also another useful source of support for patients receiving HPN. Advanced technology, standardised monitoring and a flexible approach will aid in the overall enhancement of the quality of life for patients requiring prolonged periods of nutritional support.

REFERENCES

BAPEN 1995 Enteral and parenteral nutrition in the community. A report by a Working Party of the British Association for Parenteral and Enteral Nutrition. Elia M (Chair of Working Party). BAPEN, Maidenhead
BAPEN 1995 Home parenteral nutrition: quality criteria for clinical services and the supply of nutritional fluids and equipment. Wood S (ed). BAPEN, Maidenhead.
Department of Health NHS Executive 1995 Purchasing high tech healthcare for patients at home. 17 January EL(95) 5. NHS, Leeds
Jeejeeboy KN 1983 Total parenteral nutrition in the hospital and at home. CRC Press, Boca Raton, FL, pp 1–255

FURTHER READING

ASPEN Board of Directors 1993 Guidelines for the use of parenteral and enteral nutrition in adult and paediatric patients. Journal of Parenteral and Enteral Nutrition 17(suppl):1SA–52SA
Ireton-Jones CS, Hennessy K, Howard D et al 1995 Multidisciplinary clinical care of the home parenteral nutrition patient. Infusion 1(8):21–30
Jackson MA 1983 Long term PN. British Journal of Hospital Medicine February 105–116
Mughal M, Irving MH 1986 Home parenteral nutrition in the UK and Ireland. Lancet ii:383–386
Stokes MA, Irving MH 1988 How do patients with Crohn's disease fare on home parenteral nutrition? Diseases of the Colon and Rectum 31(6): 454–458
Stokes MA, Almond DJ, Pettit SH, Mughal M, Shaffer JL, Irving MH 1988 Home parenteral nutrition: a review of 100 patient years of treatment in 76 consecutive cases. British Journal of Surgery 75:481–483

11

Living with parenteral nutrition: a patient's perspective

Steve McManus

Introduction	Practical perspective
Chronic ill health	Conclusion

INTRODUCTION

We can all expect to experience some form of illness at some time. For the majority of us illness is a short-lived experience that requires minimal to moderate social adaptation over a short period of time. This is based on a premise that acute ill health is amenable to treatment and thus a return to pre-illness social roles can be anticipated. However, for the patient requiring long-term parenteral nutrition (PN), the adaptation to illness often requires long-term changes to their social role. Their social interaction at many different interfaces such as employment, family, leisure activities can all be permanently altered often combined with devastating consequences to their self-esteem, personal self-worth and physical image. A further consideration is the fact that for those individuals requiring long-term intravenous nutrition their dependency on parenteral support is a paradox: it not only acts as their primary life support, but also acts as a constant reminder of their chronic disability.

Previous chapters have concentrated on the practical issues of managing the patient receiving PN both in hospital and at home. This chapter will provide an insight to the 'lived experience' of receiving PN and explores some of the ensuing consequences for the individual in terms of coping with chronic illness. It begins by introducing some of the broad issues around chronic ill health and the nature of PN as a therapy for chronic illness. Subsequently, using a case history and the direct testimony of a person receiving home parenteral nutrition (HPN), the theoretical issues raised regarding chronic illness will be illuminated from a practical perspective. This will aim to give the reader a three-dimensional view, not only of the complex management of this form of treatment, but also of the very real social and psychological implications for the individual.

CHRONIC ILL HEALTH

Interruption to social activity such as fulfilling employment obligations, managing a home environment, caring for children or attending a college course can legitimately be put on hold until an episode of ill health is past. However, in Western society there is growing incidence of individuals suffering some form of chronic ill health (Ferraro Donnelly 1993). Indeed, Gerhardt (1990) states that:

Modern medicine has become so successful regarding the treatment of chronic disease that prevalence rates have risen considerably in most Western countries.

The predominant reasons for this increase in prevalence are thought to be the reduction in secondary infections such as pneumonia that would previously have been a potential cause of death for the chronically ill, and the advances in drug/surgical therapy for a range of chronic illnesses (Gerhardt 1990). Conditions such as rheumatoid arthritis, multiple sclerosis (MS), AIDS, psoriasis, senile dementia, asthma and cancer have become common to the point that we all are likely to be directly aware of someone suffering from a chronic disorder. A mother with breast cancer experiencing repeated chemotherapy regimes can lead to fundamental changes in the social make-up of the family. The family unit often has to redefine internal roles. For example the children may become carers in order to allow one parent to continue with employment. When individuals accept the reality of chronic illness '… they face a long term damaging alteration to their lifestyle' (Miles 1991). This alteration is often based on the relationship between our physical self and our ability to interact with our social environment. Western culture promotes the notion of independence, self-reliance and the ability to enter reciprocal relationships with other human beings. However, consider the individual suffering from chronic heart disease who, due to persistent chronic symptoms of pain and breathlessness, becomes physically dependent on others regarding tasks previously attributable to the individual themselves. Physical dependency that requires social modification can have a devastating effect on personal self-esteem and social worth and provides a fundamental challenge to our sense of self. By nature we are social animals, and any persistent alteration to what is viewed as 'normal' function can be interpreted as aberrant behaviour and attract a degree of social stigma. Freidson (1970) states that 'a chronically ill person who "expects too much" or "makes too many demands" is likely to be rejected by society'. The social role of the chronically ill is an ambiguous one, often with their degree of social modification as a result of illness regulated by social convention.

As society's perception of health and illness alters, so does its legitimisation of chronic ill-health and the subsequent modification of a person's social roles. This raises the issue of societal awareness of certain chronic disease states and the ensuing legitimisation of the illness. Cancer is viewed by society as an unconditionally legitimate chronic disability, allowing the individual to modify or withdraw from previously identified social roles.

However, it could be argued that developments in medical technology are creating an increasing number of modern chronic disabilities that are not as yet legitimised in the broader context by society. The move to community-based care with an increasing number of previously defined 'acute' disorders being managed in this situation is drawing attention to '... the nature, effects, and experience of disabling illness' (Morgan et al 1993). Thorne & Paterson (1998) explore this trend through meta-analysis of research directed towards chronic illness experience over the past two decades. Their findings include a re-emphasis over the past 15 years through the related literature from 'client as patient to client as partner' in a move from acute secondary healthcare settings to a community-based primary care model. However, it could be suggested that this shift in emphasis for the management of chronic illness alters responsibility from the state to the individual. We have introduced the fact that chronic illness can detract from the individual's ability to enter into 'normal' social interaction and Anderson et al (1991) further state that:

Shifting the responsibility for care-taking from the state to the individual obfuscates the social context of illness and excludes the socially disadvantaged from adequate health care.

Anderson (1996) locates this movement within the current trend for individuals to take responsibility for their health and consequently for their chronic ill health. It is argued that this movement is likely to continue within Western healthcare culture as certain economic and demographic trends continue to escalate the extent of home therapies through advances in healthcare technologies:

As hospital costs increase and duration of hospital stays decrease, clients are being discharged to home care in more acute states and often with demands for high technology therapy (Smith et al 1991).

This raises the issue of 'visible' illness within society. The move towards home care and active therapy of individuals with chronic illness places the very experience of illness within the private domain. Together with the transient nature of certain chronic disabilities, this can lead to a public perception that the individual is exaggerating his experience. This compromises their withdrawal from certain aspects of social responsibility in a legitimised way. The aetiology of multiple sclerosis can lead to periods of remission and exacerbation. With the devastating physical effects of this illness often managed in the private domain, the public perception is shaped by the visible presentation of the individual only when in remission.

Nevertheless, there appears to be a paradox in this situation. Individuals living with chronic illness often become experts regarding the management of their own healthcare needs, but the domination of the biomedical model of health in Western society promotes the dependent relationship with traditional health care institutions. A founding perspective regarding

Western health culture is the functional model of health behaviour. Parsons (1951) introduced this concept in the form of 'sick role' behaviour. Illness, as stated earlier, is often related to the ability to fulfil certain social obligations. Parsons' 'sick role' acknowledges illness as a social as well as a biological state and is legitimised as long as the individual complies with certain social stipulations that surround this role. These stipulations demand willingness on the part of the individual to '... seek and co-operate with technically competent medical help' (Nettleton 1995). This emphasises the retention of control by healthcare professionals for the management of health, despite a move to community-based care and the lip service given to the concept of individual responsibility for health and ill-health management.

HOME PARENTERAL NUTRITION AS LONG-TERM THERAPY

It could be suggested that the individual requiring long-term HPN in the community experiences difficulty in the legitimisation of their disability on a variety of counts previously introduced. Home parenteral nutrition is one of the growing therapies that support the individual with chronic intestinal failure in the community. There are currently only approximately 360 individuals within the UK receiving nutritional support of this nature (Elia 1997). Much of the management of the underlying disability (intravenous nutritional support, management of stomas) occurs behind closed doors and overnight. Thus there is a poorly defined disease process at the broader public level, which is essentially invisible to public scrutiny. However, the physical, social and psychological effects of chronic intestinal illness and the consequential nutritional therapy can be every bit as devastating as the more recognised and socially legitimised chronic disabilities. Consequently this group of individuals can have a battle on two fronts: with their physical illness and with society's perception of their illness behaviour.

There appears to be extensive literature regarding the subject of chronic illness, with specific texts referring to a range of commonly attributed disease processes, as mentioned earlier. However there does not appear to be a depth of literature regarding chronic illness associated with the gastrointestinal system. Published texts focus predominantly on common bowel disorders such as ulcerative colitis and Crohn's disease (Kelly 1992). Review of the literature presented a clear paucity of information regarding the social effects of living with chronic intestinal failure combined with the need for long-term nutritional support. This is indicative of advances in technology that have created a growing number of community-based therapies with a consequential lag in social understanding regarding impact of managing this form of chronic disability in the community.

PRACTICAL PERSPECTIVE

Having introduced the concept of chronic illness in the social context, this chapter will further explore the particular impact of parenteral nutrition as a community-based therapy for chronic intestinal failure. Experiences are based on a specific case and draw on the generic findings regarding chronic illness behaviour.

Case Study 11.1

Jane (name changed for confidentiality) is a lady in her late twenties and the mother of two children who lives with her partner. During a surgical procedure after suffering a miscarriage at 16 weeks she suffered trauma to her small intestine. At the time of surgery the majority of her small intestine was removed and the remaining 30 cm attached to her large intestine. The subsequent intestinal failure, and inability of the small bowel to absorb the nutrition Jane requires, has resulted in the need for long-term intravenous nutrition in the form of PN. In the first year of receiving PN she experienced complications related to the administration of PN and required the re-insertion of a further central venous line for nutritional administration.

Jane describes her illness-related lifestyle as follows:

My life now consists of having a double-lumen Hickman line permanently inserted into the right side of my chest. I have to connect a bag of complex nutrients to this line 7 days a week. This runs through a digital pump over 10 h at night (a killer on your sex life!). It is slowed down during the last hour to wean me off and it is then disconnected. Everything is carried out under strict sterile procedure. I send a blood sample off to the hospital every week, so that the nutrients in the PN bag can be regulated to meet my body's needs. The lumens of the line have to be flushed with Hepsal regularly to prevent clotting, and the line site dressing has to be kept clean and dry. All the equipment has to be cleaned regularly. Refrigeration of the bags and expiry dates need to be checked daily.

A predominant feature of long-term disability that is specifically related to women is the feeling of guilt and personal responsibility in relation to their illness. Typically, women feel responsible for being ill and the ensuing disruption of not just their own lives, but also those of their family/social network. Despite the underlying cause of chronic ill health, men will display anger and blame fate, whilst women experience guilt and consequently hold themselves responsible not only for the social alteration in their own lives, but also that of their lay network. Jane described the destructive nature of her chronic illness as presenting a permanent and negative effect on her relationship with her children.

The bond between us that is so special ... between a mother and her children has been severed. Although you can pick up some of the pieces, things will never be the same again.

Jane indicates that it was not only the prolonged period of hospitalisation that altered the relationship with her children, but more significantly the effects of her PN treatment. The effects of chronic fatigue, the necessity of frequent hygiene measures and the sheer time demanded by managing the administration of PN at either end of the day means she has negligible time to invest in her children.

When I need to be spending quality time with my children in the evenings, I always seem to be otherwise occupied with sleeping, bathing or administering my PN bag.

As I am up so much during the night passing urine and my sleep is disturbed, it's almost impossible to get up early in the morning and help the children to prepare for school.

Woods et al (1993) introduced the concept that the effects of chronic ill health can be classified in terms of 'demands of illness'. This approach identifies that chronic illness presents certain generic demands on the individual, regardless of the underlying disease process, as well as specific demands related to the uniqueness of different chronic illnesses (Box 11.1).

Case Study 11.1 *(contd)*

Box 11.1 Demands of illness

Demands related to disease process
Physical and psychological experiences that are directly attributable to the disease process. These predominantly include symptoms such as pain, ' fatigue, nausea and weakness.

Demands related to personal disruption
These are challenges to the personal status quo and relate to issues of integrity, continuity and normalcy. These demands place an emphasis on making sense of the illness experience for the individual and his ability to adapt and monitor the bodily changes associated with the disease process.

Demands related to environmental transaction
Relationship of individual with social environment. Illness-related challenges within family relationships, local social network and healthcare providers.

Studies regarding the experience of women with chronic rheumatoid arthritis describe the individual woman's ability to develop through a transitionary period of adaptation in order eventually to gain 'mastery' over her disease. However, the concept of 'illness demand' introduced by Woods et al (1993) questions the extent or level to which mastery is achieved. Arguably Jane's experience displays a degree of mastery or adaptation over the 'disease process' demands of HPN:

There is the abdominal pain that I have learnt to adjust to quite quickly and ignore it as much as possible with the help of tablets.

However, it is evident that the demands related to environmental transaction have an extensive negative impact on her ability to cope with her disability.

My confidence has gone after the trauma that I went through and I find it hard to deal with everyday challenges now.

It could be argued that Jane's struggle with the demands related to environmental transaction stem from a loss of control over her everyday environment. Conwill (1993) states that the presence of a chronic disease process and the treatment that this may entail can lead to loss of control over patients' lives and result in ensuing expressions of helplessness.

A further manifestation of Jane's illness is the manner in which physical symptoms of her chronic disability accentuate a tangible withdrawal from previously held social activity. Pain, diarrhoea, fatigue and sweats all contribute to alter radically the pattern of Jane's life and consequently the way in which she perceives her social 'self'. The chronic nature of her symptoms, together with dependency on an abnormal approach to meeting dietary requirement, has removed a degree of control over her physical body. It is only at this point that we become aware of our dependence on the physical self to engage in society's perception of 'normal' social interaction.

Walking used to keep me fit and sane. I'd walk for miles and miles, clearing my head, just thinking. Now it's too painful and tiring.

My body can't regulate its temperature properly, which means that sometimes I sweat until I am dripping wet, especially at night. It's a really uncomfortable thing to deal with. In the summer weather it feels as though I am literally cooking sometimes, and it is not as though I can grab a cold drink or ice-lolly anymore. It's easier to stay indoors at times.

The ability to take a walk, create some private personal space or simply enjoy the summer sunshine are areas of social normality that are no longer accessible to Jane. Typically those suffering with some form of chronic illness have a mental demarcation between valued images of their past normality and the concern for their future

Case Study 11.1 (contd)

progression as a person within the context of their illness. Charmaz (cited in Nettleton 1995) describes this as an expression of 'loss of self'. In an attempt to gain some form of reconstituted self identity there can be a gradual increase in the dependence on social institutions around them. This can rapidly become a negative spiral with increasing dependency leading to a converse deconstruction of the individual's personal 'self' in terms of self-esteem, value within the social group and his sense of normality.

Stigma forms an important component regarding the manner in which individuals can interact with society from a position of chronic ill health. The very nature of diagnosis begins to formally label individuals in the context of the abnormality of their personal health. Indeed 'the identification of a stigmatising illness depends on medical diagnosis' (Morgan et al 1993). Certain diagnoses can lead to both an actual level of stigma directed towards the individual, but also the individual can create a perceived stigma around his illness. Whether the stigmatised illness is actual or perceived, it has the ability to encompass all aspects of the individual. Goffman (1963) describes this as '... the ability of a stigma to spread to the whole persona and spoil the person's identity.' Indeed, individuals can gradually be perceived in terms of their single stigmatising state. Jane, the mother of two, becomes the woman on a 'drip feed'. Thus society is able to characterise those amongst us with a chronic level of ill health and consequently attach a degree of legitimisation to their behaviour.

Jane describes herself as appearing normal, yet goes on to describe herself as a social misfit when stigmatising her inability to demonstrate an image of normality through tolerating a 'normal' diet. Diet and the way we manage our daily nutritional intake is hugely significant in Western culture. Food and its impact on our social fabric are firmly linked on a number of fronts. Our day and consequent interaction with family, friends and work associates is linked to meal requirement as a social opportunity as well as a physical necessity. Meal times may be the main opportunity for families to spend time together, courtship often occurs over 'dinner for two', and there is an entire industry dedicated to physical health based on diet. If the ability to interact through a recognised social mechanism is removed, then both actual and perceived stigma can develop in relation to that individual's limiting factor.

Jane also describes the stigmatising effect of physical appearance. She describes a state of disfigurement.

The scarring probably affects me more than anything else. Everybody is vain in their own little ways but as I was always very slim and figure conscious, this really gets me. I'm on my third line [central venous catheter] now and that is six sets of scars on my upper chest, there is the scar along my stomach and some small scars on my neck due to intravenous catheters inserted during surgery. Sometimes I feel like a freak.

The vision of the perfect physical form is constantly available and reinforced through social channels such as product advertising, television and film imagery. This shapes and dictates both the individual and societal view of normal and abnormal appearance. Physical disfigurement such as facial scarring due to burns or extensive visible birthmarks can attract a range of stigmatising behaviour from simple avoidance of the individual through to blatant discrimination such as the inability to secure employment that has a level of public interface. Jane verbalises this perceived level of stigma regarding her physical appearance and emphasises the value she placed on her physical appearance prior to the development of her illness. This further demonstrates the impact of 'loss of self' that occurs through the progression of chronic illness as alteration in personal image from the pre-illness state is steadily reinforced.

CONCLUSION

This chapter has identified the use of PN as treatment for a chronic health disorder. The experience of living with this treatment is explored in terms of the major physical, social and psychological effects that patients experience as a result of this continuous and highly invasive consequence of their illness. Health professionals involved in the home care of this group of patients (or indeed considering the use of this therapy even on a short-term in-patient basis) need to recognise the impact that this therapy can have on the individual. An understanding of the life of the chronically ill patient in the community can assist healthcare practitioners to '… gauge the intended as well as unintended effects of clinical measures' (Gerhardt 1990). Parenteral nutrition adds to the growing number of treatments that are able to support community-based care. The evidence is that this trend is likely to increase, not decrease. It is vital that the very real effect of managing chronic intestinal failure is understood by healthcare staff.

The impact of a disease or treatment on the patient as person, i.e. his identity, may be an aspect widely neglected in modern clinical practice. (Gerhardt 1990)

Only this level of understanding will allow the necessary psychological support and adaptation to commence before the individual is faced with the prospect of managing PN in the home.

REFERENCES

Anderson JM, Blue C, Lau A 1991 Women's perspectives on chronic illness: ethnicity, ideology and restructuring of life. Social Science in Medicine 33(2):101–113
Anderson JM 1996 Empowering patients: issues and strategies. Social Science in Medicine 43(5):697–705
Conwill J 1993 Understanding and combating helplessness. Rehabilitation Nursing 18(6):388–394
Elia M (ed) 1997 The 1997 Annual Report of the British Artificial Nutrition Survey (BANS). BAPEN, Maidenhead
Ferraro Donnelly G 1993 Chronicity: concept and reality. Holistic Nursing Practice 8(1):1–7
Freidson E 1970 The profession of medicine. Aldine, New York
Gerhardt U 1990 Qualitative research on chronic illness: the issue and the story. Social Science in Medicine 30(11):1149–1159
Goffman E 1963 Stigma: notes on the management of a spoiled identity. Prentice Hall, Englewood Cliffs, NJ
Kelly M 1992 Colitis. Routledge, London
Miles A 1991 Women, health and medicine. Open University Press, Buckingham
Morgan M, Calnan M, Manning N 1993 Sociological approaches to health and medicine. Routledge, London
Nettleton S 1995 The sociology of health and illness. Polity, Cambridge
Parsons T 1951 The social system. Free Press, Glencoe
Smith CE, Giefer CK, Bieker L 1991 Technological dependency: a preliminary model and pilot of home parenteral nutrition. Journal of Community Health Nursing 8(4):245–254
Thorne S, Paterson B 1998 Shifting images of chronic illness. Image: Journal of Nursing Scholarship 30(2):173–178
Woods NF, Habernam MR, Packard NJ 1993 Demands of illness and individual, dyadic, and family adaptation in chronic illness. Western Journal of Nursing Research 15(1):10–30

12

Conclusion

Katherine Fermo

Introduction
The multidisciplinary approach to PN
The role of the clinical nurse specialist
Basic competencies

Maintenance of the patient on PN
Benefits of the NST
Conclusion

INTRODUCTION

Nourishment is essential for life, and correct nutrition is necessary to sustain health. The average human being can survive for 7–10 days without fluids and will die without food after 50–70 days. From birth humans are encouraged to eat for growth, healing and a sense of wellbeing. Nutrition is the very basis of life and survival, having many social symbolic, cultural and religious connotations that must be addressed in patient care. Eating is usually associated with great affection, whereas withholding food can be associated with punishment.

Parenteral nutrition (PN) provides life-sustaining therapy for those who are unable, for one reason or another, to consume adequate nutrition enterally (via the gut), and as such are at risk of developing the debilitating complications of malnutrition. These complications include a greater susceptibility to infection, delayed recovery from illness and surgery, and an increased likelihood of death. For these reasons, PN has become a necessity for selected patients experiencing intestinal failure, both in the hospital and community setting.

This book has examined the ways in which the best outcome can be achieved for the patient receiving PN, from the initial assessment to long-term maintenance of feeding therapy. The issues of patient preparation and education have been covered, as well as choice of catheter, method of insertion, and ways of managing PN. Ultimately, the success of long-term PN depends on the skill and commitment of the healthcare professionals involved in patient care.

THE MULTIDISCIPLINARY APPROACH TO PN

The principles and importance of early nutritional assessment have been discussed by various disciplines. It has become evident that a combination of clinical and biochemical assessment can predict, with reasonable success, patients who may be at risk of malnutrition-associated complications. On the basis of this information, obtained from a direct and collaborative multidisciplinary approach, valid clinical outcomes become evident. These include improved survival, fewer clinical complications and reduced hospital admission.

Nutrition and the detrimental effects of malnutrition are too important to be the sole responsibility of a single member of the health team. The adequate provision of clinical nutrition requires input from a variety of specialised providers. These may be people working together as a Nutrition Support Team (NST) or Nutrition Support Committee (NSC), or may be individuals with a direct responsibility and interest in artificial nutrition. The multidisciplinary team usually consists of medical, nursing, dietetics and pharmacological representation.

Hindle et al (1996) and Fisher & Opper (1996) are among a handful of researchers who provide evidence suggesting that the use of the multidisciplinary team in nutritional assessment and support has fundamental potential benefits. These benefits present themselves in the form of reduced catheter-related infections, reduced overall costs, improved patient recovery and prompt hospital discharge. A survey conducted in 1991 revealed that only 32.5% of hospitals in the UK had established a NST (Payne-James et al 1992, cited in Hindle et al 1996 p. 61).

Following prompt and appropriate nutritional assessment, health team members are able to implement adequate and effective nutrition for their patients. This is essential for both comprehensive management and prevention of disease. The effective management of the patient requiring artificial nutrition necessitates detailed evaluation of gut function, nutritional status and, ultimately, the interaction of the nutritional state and the clinical course of treatment.

Fisher & Opper (1996) reveal that significant differences in complication rates exist between patients receiving PN monitored by a NST and those monitored by individual physicians. Nehme (1980) supports these findings, suggesting that nutritional support provided by medical teams only has significantly higher complication rates associated with cvc placement, as well as higher rates of PN-related metabolic complications. The provision of daily monitoring of biochemical values and the routine interdisciplinary clinical bedside rounds enable the NST to identify and significantly reduce the possible metabolic abnormalities and catheter-related complications that may be associated with PN.

Appropriate patient selection is just as important as the safe provision and early detection of PN-related complications. The NST provides a resource that can accurately assess and implement the appropriate route of nutritional administration required on an individual basis. Twomey (1993) found that in 1992 and 1993 only 59% of PN requested by medical teams alone received this form of nutrition.

The presence of a NST is clearly not always possible. However, a designated person responsible for the provision of nutrition, generally a dietitian, will identify inappropriate candidates and will be able to recommend enteral nutrition as an alternative, thus reducing significantly the cost of nutritional administration via the central venous route.

The literature cited above suggests that the development and maintenance of a NST will reflect fewer complications associated with the administration of PN, improved patient care, and therefore clear beneficial economic results.

THE ROLE OF THE CLINICAL NURSE SPECIALIST

Previous chapters have illustrated the value of a nurse specialising within the field of artificial nutrition. The role of the clinical nurse specialist (CNS) within the NST is directly linked with the preinsertion, insertion and postinsertion care of cvcs in patients receiving PN. In addition to this, the ward-based nurse provides a vital link between the patient and other members of the healthcare team.

The nurse, ward-based or specialist, is the person best placed to know how a patient is reacting to a disease process and to the received therapy she is receiving. It is through regular liaisons with the nursing staff at ward level, who are in continuous contact with the patient, that the NST is made aware of any physiological and psychological functions that may reflect on the alteration and administration of PN. The CNS and the ward nurses are in an ideal position to evaluate the effectiveness of PN. They will be instrumental in the safe delivery of PN and are usually the first to witness adverse reactions.

The method by which PN is administered is often determined by the quality of available venous access. However, owing to advances in the manufacture of catheters, central venous access can now successfully be gained by using a peripheral approach in addition to the central method of administering PN. However, peripheral veins often do not withstand the indefinite administration of some PN components, and long term PN usually requires access to a central vein. It is at this point that the specific role of the CNS within the NST varies from that of the nurse at ward level. Studies have shown that the presence or absence of a CNS strongly affects the incidence of catheter-related sepsis.

Much of the literature reviewed clearly highlights the importance of the NST in reducing the incidence of catheter-related sepsis, a role which can be largely attributable to the CNS. Sanders & Sheldon (1986, cited in Murphy & Lipman 1987 p. 196) highlight the results of a study on catheter-related sepsis with and without the combined input of NSTs. It was found that catheter-related sepsis associated with PN without the input and influences of the NST was 28.6%, while with the direct involvement of NSTs, catheter-related sepsis fell dramatically to 4.7%.

In some instances, the role of the CNS within the NST has been extended to encompass that of catheter inserter. Hamilton (1995 p. 39) highlights the added benefits to the extended role of the CNS within the field of PN (Box 12.1). Although the insertion of the cvc is associated with an increased exposure to life-threatening complications, an efficient and honed technique can significantly reduce the incidence of procedural complications. The adoption of the CNS with catheter insertion skills by the NST provides not only expert skills associated with catheter insertion, but also continuity of care to those patients requiring PN. Clearly, it is beneficial if a dedicated operator is available to gain central venous access for PN, but this is not always possible. A compromise may include the use of a standard device inserted surgically, attracting a high standard of aseptic technique and therefore reducing the risk of complications associated with catheter insertion. Another alternative is the peripherally inserted central catheter (PICC), which may also attract fewer complications associated with insertion. Continuity can then be guaranteed in the insertion and subsequent management of the catheter.

The role of the CNS within the NST has been shown to reduce significantly catheter-related complications, as well as improving the quality of care administered to those patients receiving PN. Functioning within the ideal conditions imposed by NSTs, through the assessment, planning, implementation and evaluation of strict procedure and protocol, PN can have an enormous therapeutic potential. Administration and supervision of PN by experienced personnel adhering to strict protocol often results in fewer complications, enhanced patient care, and both therapeutic and economic benefits.

Box 12.1   The benefits of extending the role of a CNS within the NST team

- A short response time is offered
- Frequency of central line placement and experience of continued practice ensures minimal complications
- A dedicated team approach to central venous cannulation results in a significant reduction in infection rates
- Protocols for the management of cvcs encourages quality of patient care
- CNS liaison regarding management of cvcs
- Reduced costs associated with no theatre and anaesthetic time
- Training opportunities for medical staff
- Medical staff are free to perform other urgent duties
- Ward-based procedure reducing patient anxiety associated with familiarity of staff
- The CNS counsels and provides in-depth information to the patient prior to the insertion of the cvc. This facilitates a holistic approach by the CNS
- Assessment and provision of analgesia and sedation by the CNS throughout the procedure
- The CNS identifies and promptly treats possible complications associated with central venous cannulation
- Provides ongoing education and liaises regularly with nurses and staff at ward level regarding the identification and treatment of possible catheter-related complications

BASIC COMPETENCIES

From the time of the Second World War, intravenous therapy has gradually shifted from the medical to the nursing domain. These changes have been driven to some extent by staff shortages, but are also a clear reflection of the nursing profession's willingness to develop and engage in extended practices. Since the development and release of *The Scope of Professional Practice* (UKCC 1992), nurses have been afforded the opportunity to participate in newly developing nurse specialist roles. These include central venous cannulation, providing an integral role within NSTs and more recently, nurse prescribing. For this climate to continue, basic principles and competencies for the maintenance and ongoing success of these programmes must be established (Scales 1997).

For those patients receiving alimentation via cvcs, nurses, medical staff and other healthcare professionals must be equipped with an adequate understanding of the possible complications associated with this route of nutrition and its metabolic complications, as well as the ability to act appropriately upon these complications, should they occur. Increasingly the responsibilities for the insertion and care of cvcs for the administration of PN are becoming integral within the extended role of nursing practice.

Central venous catheterisation for the administration of PN should, in principle, be a relatively easy and consistent procedure. However, the human venous system is extremely variable, and therefore often presents the operator with many challenging difficulties. Where anatomy and venous structure remains reasonably constant, there is still a considerable risk of injury to vital structures. For these reasons, concise, accurate and efficient patient assessment and the utilisation of experienced operators significantly reduces unnecessary complications. Competent catheter insertion and specialised care of cvcs post insertion is rapidly becoming an integral part of the clinical evaluation of hospitalised and community-based patients. With the emphasis placed currently on community-based acute healthcare, appropriate education in the care of patients receiving PN in the community is essential. No doubt the future will see many more intravenous therapies delivered in the community. Providing the expertise is available, this will enhance patient care and enable families to receive community-based care.

MAINTENANCE OF THE PATIENT ON PN

The initial enthusiasm for the use of PN was tempered somewhat by the incidence of therapy-related complications. These complications have been classified as mechanical, metabolic or septic abnormalities. According to Dalton et al (1984), the most common cause of these phenomena was the inadequate provision of patient monitoring. The development of multidisciplinary teams to manage PN was advocated to overcome these problems. Many institutions have developed NSTs to assume primary responsibility for managing all patients receiving PN.

Owing to the complexity of intestinal failure and the subsequent introduction of PN, the Department of Health has recognised the need for specialised units to manage patients requiring PN. Biochemical issues can often be coupled with vascular access difficulties, and a specialist unit can provide the necessary advice and expertise to another centre with less exposure to PN.

If a ward or NST is to function efficiently and successfully, thorough education programmes relating to PN and frameworks for supervision must be clearly implemented. The ongoing education, training and re-training for all personnel involved in patient care and the constitution, administration and maintenance of PN is vital if patients are to complete therapy in the absence of associated complications.

It is desirable that the objectives and functions of the NST are properly defined. These can be periodically and systematically assessed, revealing areas or techniques that require improvement in safety and efficacy. All members of the NST must be able to contribute the expertise of their own discipline whilst respecting and recognising the priorities and responsibilities of others. Each role within the team provides an invaluable clinical source of information for other participating members. The physician's detailed and extensive knowledge of disease processes, supported by the clinical expertise of the other members, namely the dietitian, pharmacist and clinical nurse specialist, provide a framework through which accurate nutritional assessment can be made. Hamaoui (1987 p. 418) states that within NSTs each participating member of the team should possess 'sufficient basic knowledge in these subjects to enable them to apply their own discipline's expertise intelligently and usefully'.

Success in the treatment of intestinal failure using PN will be demonstrated by a cohesive and effective multidisciplinary approach, with each member as important as the next in the provision of this complex and expensive method of nutrition.

BENEFITS OF THE NST

From a managerial point of view, it is necessary to provide evidence for the benefits derived from the provision of a NST (or NSC). It is important that the institution of care (the NHS) is clearly able to determine whether the benefits of the NST are worth the investment in time and money. Therefore, it becomes pertinent to argue for the development and instigation of a NST in the most cost-effective way. It can be argued, as has been shown in the literature, that the management of clinical nutrition by a multidisciplinary team significantly improves patient care and outcome,

---

Box 12.2   Economic commitments and advantages associated with the NST

Economic commitments
- Development of the NST
- Ongoing costs of the NST
- Possible increase in expenditure on nutritional materials and
- Ancillary equipment and services

Advantages
- Standardisation of regimens
- Accurate identification of 'at-risk' patients
- Reduction of medical complications
- Implementation of cost-effective choices for nutritional support
- Reduced workload for ward staff
- Minimisation of waste
- Purchasing efficiency
- Reduction in length of patient stay
- Reduction in 'bed blocking'
- Reduction in admission waiting times

---

thus representing the most cost-effective alternative for the provision of nutritional support in hospitals (Hindle et al 1996). Box 12.2 highlights the advantages and economic consequences of establishing a NST (Hindle et al 1996 p. 64).

Unfortunately, financial constraints do not allow all senior managers to support this theory, and it is in this situation that an awareness and commitment to nutrition from ward-based nurses can identify the malnourished patient and supplementation can begin.

In the preparation of a business case for the establishment of a nutrition team, the previous points provide a compelling argument. It has been suggested by a significant amount of research that the mobilisation of NSTs within the hospital setting serves to accurately identify appropriate referrals and provide cost-effective measures related to the administration of PN.

CONCLUSION

When researching and gathering literature on the administration and care of patients receiving PN, it becomes clear that the prolonged maintenance of these patients, typically receiving PN via cvcs, has historically been a limiting factor. This book has examined the necessity for accurate and effective patient identification and assessment, and has highlighted the importance of implementation and ongoing care of patients receiving PN.

The use of specialised NSTs involved in all aspects of the delivery of PN has been shown to significantly reduce the incidence of PN-related complications associated with mechanical, clinical and biochemical abnormalities. A collaborative effort from healthcare personnel involved and participating actively within the NST or NSC will aid in avoiding inappropriate patient selection and management, thus promoting an efficient and cost-effective service.

REFERENCES

Dalton MJ, Schepers G, Gee JP, Alberts CC, Eckhauser FE, Kirking DM 1984 Consultative total parenteral nutrition teams: the effect on the incidence of total parenteral nutrition-related complications. Journal of Parenteral and Enteral Nutrition 8(2):146–152

Fisher GG, Opper FH 1996 An interdisciplinary nutrition support team improves quality of care in a teaching hospital. Journal of the American Dietetic Association 96(2):176–178

Hamilton HC 1995 Central lines inserted by clinical nurse specialists. Nursing Times 91(17):38–39

Hamaoui E 1987 Assessing the Nutrition Support Team. Journal of Parenteral and Enteral Nutrition 11(4):412–421

Hindle T, Dhoot R, Georgieva C 1996 Clinical nutrition in NHS hospitals. British Journal of Intensive Care February:61–65

Murphy LM, Lipman TO 1987 Central venous catheter care in parenteral nutrition: a review. Journal of Parenteral and Enteral Nutrition 11(2):190–199

Nehme AE 1980 Nutritional support of the hospitalised patient. Journal of the American Medical Association 243(19):1906–1908

Scales K 1997 Practical and professional aspects of IV therapy. Professional Nurse Supplement 12(8):S3–S5

Twomey PL 1993 Cost effectiveness of nutritional support. In: Rombeau JL, Caldwell M D (eds) Clinical nutrition parenteral nutrition, 2nd edn. WB Saunders, Philadelphia, pp 401–408

UKCC (1992) The scope of professional practice. UKCC, London

Index

*Numbers in **bold** refer to tables or illustrations*

A

Abdominal pain, 150
Acetone, skin defatting, 160, 190
Acquired immune deficiency syndrome
(AIDS), 45–46
home parenteral nutrition (HPN), 15
mucositis, 35
Activated partial thromboplastin time
(APTT), 103
Administration sets, changing, 163
Advantages and disadvantages
enteral nutrition, 37
parenteral nutrition, 37
peripheral parenteral nutrition (PPN), 51
Advocacy, CNS role, 21
Air embolism, 129, 196–197
Albumin
concentrations, 10
supplementation, 202
Alcohol intake, 33
Alcohol-based
cleansing solutions, 190
handwashes, 159
Alcoholic patients, 178
magnesium deficiency, 5
Allergy assessment, 106
Ambulatory infusion pumps, 56, 213
Amino acids, 4, 6
excessive administration, neonates, 14
peripheral route administration, 50
Anaphylactic shock, **149**
Antacids, 178
Anthropometric measurements, 34, 140,
145, **146**
Antibacterial/antiseptic handwash, 158, 159
Antibiotics
catheter-related sepsis, 12, 158
preoperative, 96
topical, 160
Antithrombin 3 deficiency, 13
Anxiety, 83, 89–91, 94, 102
about body image, 153
needle phobia, 91
transition to enteral feeding, 154

Apathy, 32
Appetite, 154, 183
Arginine, 6
Arrhythmias
before CVC insertion, 103–104
post procedural, 123, 124, 125, 126, 133, 141
refeeding syndrome, 179
Arterial puncture, 127
Asepsis, training HPN patients, 210
Aseptic service unit (ASU), 175
Assessment, 9, 102–106, 139–140
allergies, 106
of anxiety, 90–91
cardiovascular function, 103–104
clinical, 102
dietetic, 174–176
gastrointestinal function, 35–36, 39, 52
HPN patients
home assessment, 214–215
psychological assessment, 206
training suitability, 207, 209
laboratory, 103
neurological function, 105–106
nutritional, 31-35, 39, 51, 106
parenteral versus enteral nutrition, 36–38
algorithm, **38**
patient's information requirements, 88
peripheral parenteral nutrition, 47–51
respiratory function, 104–105
specific disease processes, 39–47
vascular function, 105
Audible alarm, infusion pump, 197
Audit, CNS responsibility, 21–22
Axillary vein 61

B

Back pain, 124
Bacterial/toxin translocation, 1, 6, 173
Barrier to infection, intestine as, 1
Baseline measurements, 9, 139–140
Basilic veins, 50, 60, 61, 75
Bed, checking function, 97
Bedside nutritional assessment, 31–35, 39, 51
how to perform, 32–35
reasons for performing, 32
summary, 33

Benzodiazepines, 91
Biliary sludge, 14, 202
Biochemist, **19**
Biomedical model, domination, 221
Blood
    analysis, 10, 96–97
        monitoring blood sugar, 9, 42, 146,
            149–150, 178
        viewing results, 97–98
    obtaining cultures, 12, 188
    recognising venous/arterial, 120
Blood pressure, 9
Blood products, administration, 96–97, 195
Bodily fluids, electrolyte content, **175**
Body image, 58, 93–94, 153
    case study, 75
Body mass index (BMI), 34
    interpretation, **176**
Bone marrow transplantation, 44
    dressings, 191
    multilumen catheters, 70
Booklets, 87, 207
Bowel rest, 43
Bra straps, 93
Brachial plexus damage, 129
Branched-chain-enriched amino acid
        solutions, 6
British Association of Parenteral and
        Enteral Nutrition (BAPEN), 28, 87
    clinical benefits of NST/NSC, 25
    LITRE group, 214
    preparing patient for HPN, **208–209**
        district nurses, 210
        Learning Goals booklet, 207
        patient skills at discharge, 216
    standard for supply of PN and
        equipment, 216
Broviac catheters, 211
Budget, CNS responsibility, 22
Burns, 46

C

Cachexia, 44
Calories
    assessing requirement, 175
    effects of overfeeding, 179–180
    hypocaloric feeding, 11
Cancer, 44–45, 220
    home parenteral nutrition (HPN), 15
Candida infections, 12, 156
Cannulae, peripheral parenteral nutrition,
        8, 49, 65
    see also Catheters
Carbohydrates, administration, 50
    overfeeding, 179–180
Carbon dioxide production, increased, 199
Cardiac murmurs, 12

Cardiac tamponade, 126, 129
Cardiovascular system
    assessment, prior CVC insertion, 103–104
    monitoring
        patients on PN, 141
        postpercutaneous CVC insertion, 124
Carotid artery, puncture, 127
Catheter hub
    care of, 162–163
    infection, 188
Catheters
    choosing appropriate, 55–80
        available products, 8, 49, 68–71, 165,
            166, 188
        case studies, 71–80
        catheters and sites, **60**
        clinical issues and potential
            complications, 56–57
        insertion of CVC, 63–68, 109–113
        patient considerations, 57–58
        patients with needle phobia, 91
        purpose and duration of therapy, 56
        suitable vein availability, 58–63
    guidelines for management, 154–170
        catheter damage, 13, 170, 195
        catheter occlusion, 165–170, 191–195
        catheter-related sepsis, 155–164
            see also Infection, catheter-related
        nursing care, 160–163
    see also Central venous catheters (CVC);
        Peripherally inserted central
        catheters (PICC)
Central parenteral nutrition (CPN), 8, 14
    definition, 2
Central venous catheters (CVC)
    complications *see* Damage to catheter;
        Infection, catheter-related;
        Occlusion, catheter
    insertion, 56, 63–68, 101–134
        by clinical nurse specialist, 68, 230, 231
        discussion, 133–134
        equipment available, 67, 68, 116
        indications, 101
        method, factors influencing choice,
            113–116
        patient assessment and information,
            102–106
        percutaneous, infraclavicular
            approach, 116–129
        PICC insertion, 129–133
            see also Peripherally inserted central
            catheters (PICC)
        techniques, 64–67, 109–113
    preparation for insertion, 83–99, 106–109
        aims, 83–86
        case study, 99
        helpful hints, 97–98
        patient concerns, 57–58, 89–95
        patient preparation, 106–107, 118

Central venous catheters (CVC) (*contd*)
  practical requirements, 95–97
  preparation of operating venue and
    equipment, 107–109
  provision of information, 86–89
Central venous thrombosis (CVT), 12–13,
    164, 191–193
  predisposing factors, 164–165
  prevention and treatment, 165, 193
    unblocking catheter, 193–194
  signs and symptoms, 165
Cephalic veins, 50, 60, 61, 75
Cerebral thrombosis, 126
Chest X-ray
  catheter occlusion, 169
    fibrin flap, **192**
  CVC post-insertion, 9, 124, **125**
    misplaced catheters, 127
  pneumothorax, 126, 127, **128**, 196
Chest drain, 196
Chest pain, 127, 196, 197
Children, 31, 58
  bone marrow transplantation, 44
    see also Bone marrow transplantation
  as carers, 220
  copper deficiency, 201–202
  gallstones, 150
  head circumference, 34
  height and weight, 34
  inflammatory bowel disease, 43
  paediatric CNS, 20
  relationship with, patients on HPN, 223
Chlorhexidine, 159, 160, 190
Cholecystitis, 202
Cholestasis, 14, 173, 202
Cholesterol, monitoring, 180
Chronic ill health, 219–222
Clavicular site, sutures, 122, 123, 161, 162
Clean room, HPN patients, 214
Cleasing solutions, 159, 160, 189, 190
Clinical benefits of NST/NSC, 25
Clinical condition
  assessing, 33–35, 102
  method of CVC insertion, 113–114
  monitoring, 9, 141–146
Clinical nurse specialist (CNS), **19**, 20–22,
    27, 229–230
Clinical role
  clinical nurse specialist (CNS), 21
  pharmacist, 23–24
Clinimix, 174
Clippers, 95
Closed Luer lock connection devices,
    162–163
Coagulopathy, accepted parameters, 103
Code of Professional Practice, UKCC, 138
Cold, sensitivity to, 35
Collateral venous distribution, chest wall, 165
Coma, hyperosmolar, **148**

Commercial companies, home delivery PN
    and equipment, 215–216
Communication
  barriers to effective, 85–86
  NST/NSC team members, 27
  reducing anxiety, 90–91
Community nursing team, 88
  intravenous nurse specialist, 193
Competencies, basic, 231
Compliance, 57
Complications, 10–14, 56–57, 141–142,
    187–204, 231–232
  air embolism, 129, 196–197
  associated with PN
    long-term, 150–151
    short-term, 147–150
  avoiding, 133
  catheter-related
    catheter damage, 13, 170, 195
    occlusions, 13, 50, 51, 165–170, 191–195
    sepsis, 9, 11–12, 114, 129, 150, 154,
      155–164, 187–191
  equipment, 197–198
  haemorrhage, 124, 127, 195
  HPN patients, 212, 217
  nutritional, 11, 178–181
  patient complications, 198–203
  percutaneous CVC insertion, 126–129
  PICC insertion, 132–133
  pneumothorax, 124, 126, 127–128, 142,
    195–196
  rates of, differences in, 228
Compounding nutrient solutions, 6–7, 24
Concomitant medications, 199
Congestive cardiac failure, 182
Conscious state, monitoring, 123
Consent, 84–85, 97
Consultant clinician, 19–20
Contamination, PN bags, 163, 188
Continuous infusion, 7
Contraindications, CVC insertion, 104
Copper deficiency, 201–202
Costs of HPN, health authority acceptance,
    215–216
Cough, 124, 126, 196
Counselling, 75, 153
Crohn's disease, 205
  case studies
    Port-a-Cath insertion, 74–77
    preparation for CVC insertion, 99
    tunnelled silicone CVC insertion, 78–80
  elemental diets, 43
  magnesium deficiency, 5
  trace element and vitamin screening, 178
  see also Short bowel syndrome
Current venous access sites, 114
Cyanosis, 197
Cyclical PN, 7, 8, 151–152, 153, 154, 180–181,
    183

Cyclical PN (*Contd*)
  heparinising catheter 166
  HPN patients 217
Cytokines, 3

D

Dacron cuffs, 8, 61, 120, 122, 162
  low infection rate, 188
  position, 12, 121
Damage to catheters, 13, 170, 195
Defatting skin, 160, 190
Definitions, 2
Delayed pneumothorax, 128
Delays, avoiding, 89–90
Delivery system, 163–164
Demands of illness, 223, 224
Dependency, 220, 225
Depilatory cream, 95
Depression
  HPN patients, 206
  weight loss, 32
Dietetic aspects, 173–185
  assessing appropriateness of referral,
    173–174
  dietetic assessment, 174–176
  dietetic monitoring, 176–178
  nutritional complications of PN, 178–181
  weaning off PN, 181–184, 185
Dietician, **19**, 22–23, 229
  nutritional requirement calculation, 140
  transition to enteral/oral feeding, 154
District nursing team, HPN patients,
    209–210, 216
Diuretics, 178, 199
Documentation, 89
  of complications, 193
Doppler device, vein identification, 61
Double-lumen cuffed catheter, **79**
Dress preferences, 92–93, 94
Dressings, 160–161, 189, 190–191
  PICC, **132**
  pressure, 127, 195
Drip stands, 153
  HPN patients, 213
Drug intake, 33
Drug-nutrient interactions, 23–24
Dynamometry, 10, 144–145
Dysphagia, 35
Dyspnoea, 127, 196, 197, 217

E

Economic commitments and advantages of
    NST, 233
Education
  HPN patients, 207–210

of personnel, 232
role of
  clinical nurse specialist, 20–21, 86, 94
  dietician, 23
  pharmacist, 24
Educational benefits of NST/NSC
    expertise, 26
Elastomeric hydrogel catheters, **69**
Elderly patients, sedation, 106, 123–124
Electrolytes, 5
  burns patients, 46
  content, intravenous replacement fluids,
    175
  effect on lipid emulsion stability, 6–7
  imbalance, 11, **148**, 175, 203
  measuring, 9–10, 146
Elemental diets, Crohn's disease, 43
Emergency situation, 104
End stage disease, cancer, 44–45
Endoluminal brushing, 12
Energy, 4
Engorgement, upper limbs and neck veins
  CVT symptoms, 165
  Trendelenburg position, 98
Enteral nutrition, 2, 36, 52, 173, 174
  advantages and disadvantages, 37
  burns patients, 46–47
  gastrointestinal surgery, 42
  restricted intake, 152
  short bowel syndrome, 40
  transition to, 7, 23, 154, 181–184
Enterococcal infection, 156
Environmental transaction, illness
    demands, 224
Equipment
  available, 67, 68, 116
  complications, 197–198
  HPN patients, 213–214, 215
    delivery, 215–216
Essential fatty acids, 4
  deficiency, 200–201
Ethanol flush, 13, 170, 194
Exit-site, 87
  cleansing, 160
  infections, 12, 156, 189
  monitoring, 160
  oozing, 127
  suturing, 122–123, 132
External jugular vein, 62
Extracellular slime, 156
Eyes, examination, 34

F

Family, redefining roles, 220
Farwell report, 163
Fatty infiltration of liver, 151, 180, 202
Fear of procedure, 89–90

Feedback, patient understanding, 89
Femoral vein, 62–63, 75
  infection risk, 92
  privacy issues, 93
Fibrin
  deposits, 165
    treatment, 169–170
  flap formation, 192
  sheath formation, 155–156, 164, 166
Filters, 7, 50, 163
Financial issues
  benefits of NST/NSC, 25–26
  cost implications, HPN, 206
Fine-bore catheters, 8, 49, 166
Fingers, tingling, 126, 129
Fistulae, 43–44
  case study, silicone catheter CVC
    insertion, 78–80
  high-output, 5, 9, 147
Fluids, 5
  burns patients, 46
  fluid balance
    chart, 9
    monitoring, 142–144, 176–177
Flushing catheters, 13, 166–167, 170, 193, 194
  detection of occlusion, 169
Food, recording intake
  charts, 154
  diaries, 33
Fresh frozen plasma, 97
Full blood count, 96, 97
Fullness, feeling of, 154

G

Gall bladder stasis, 14, 173, 202
Gallstones, 150, 202
Gastric emptying, 182–183
Gastrointestinal system
  cell turnover, 182
  fistulae see Fistulae
  function, 1, 6
    assessment, 35–36, 39, 52
  intestinal failure, 1, 13, 15
  surgery, 42–43
    see also Small bowel: resection
Gauze dressings, 160, 190, 191
Gender, attitudes to PN, 223
General monitoring and observation, 145, 146
Gloves, use of, 119, 159
Glucose
  administration
    excessive, 4, 14
    thrombosis risk, 13
  intolerance, **149**, 198–199
  maximum oxidation, 180
  monitoring blood levels, 9, 146, 149–150, 178

in pancreatitis, 42
Glutamine, 6
Glyceryl trinitrate (GTN) patches, 8, 51, 67, 133
Glycosuria, 198
GP
  emergency contact, HPN patients, 212
  written information about HPN, 216
Groshong single-lumen PICC, **66**
Gums, examination, 34

H

Haematocrit, 146
Haemoglobin concentration, 146
Haemorrhage, 124, 127, 195
Haemothorax, 128–129
Hair
  observation, 34
  removal, 95
Hand grip dynamometry, 10, 144–145
Handrubs, alcohol, 159
Handwashing, 158–159
Head circumference, measuring, 34
Head injured patients, 105
Health authority, confirmation of cost
    acceptance, HPN patients, 215–216
Height measurement, 34, 121
Heparin
  addition to PN solution, 8, 13, 51, 165, 166
  coating catheters, 70, 166
  flushing catheters, 166, 167, 193
  heparin lock, 167
  solution destabilisation, 7
Hepatobiliary system, effect of PN, 13, 14
  see also Liver
Hickman-type catheters, 78, 188, 211
History taking, 33
Holidays, 95
Home parenteral nutrition (HPN), 14–15, 139, 205–218
  anxiety, 90
  catheter considerations, 58, 59
    size, 70
  CNS role, 20–21
  coming to terms with, 93–94, 205–207
  discharge, 215–216
    education, patients/carers prior to, 207–210
  equipment required, 213–214
  home assessment, 214–215
  information booklets, 87
  as long-term therapy, 222
    patient's perspective, case study, 223–225
  monitoring, 9, 11
    and complications, 216–217
  social aspects, 94–95
  training programme, 210–212

Home parenteral nutrition (HPN) (*contd*)
Huber needles, **76**
Hydration status, observation, 34
Hydrocortisone, addition to PN solution, 8, 51
Hydrogen peroxide, 190
Hyperammonaemia, 201
Hyperemesis gravidarum, 47
Hyperglycaemia, 4, 9, 11, **148**, 198, 199
   HPN patients, 217
Hypermagnesaemia, 200
Hyperosmolar coma, **148**
Hyperosmolar solution, CVT formation, 164
Hypoalbuminaemia, 202–203
Hypocalcaemia, 5
Hypocaloric feeding, 11
Hypoglycaemia, 182, 199
   rebound, 11, **148**
Hypokalaemia, 5
Hypomagnesaemia, 200
Hypophosphataemia, 5, 11, **148**, 199–200
Hypotension, 124
Hypotonic fluids, restricting intake, 184
Hypovolaemic patients, 104

I

Ileocaecal valve, 40
Immunosuppressed patients, 92, 189
Indications, parenteral nutrition, 2–3
Infection, catheter-related, 9, 11–12, 92, 114, 129, 150, 154, 155–164, 187–191
   CNS role, retrieving blood cultures, 21
   detection/diagnosis, 156–158, 188–189
   guidelines for HPN patients, 212, 217
   main contaminants, 156
   pathophysiology, 155–156
   prevention, 189–191
   protocol for management, **157**
   reduction in, CNS/NST involvement in care, 25, 26, 229
   sites of infection, 188
      insertion sites, 92
Inflammatory bowel disease, 43
   fistulae, 44
   hepatobiliary disease development, 14
   see also Crohn's disease; Ulcerative colitis
Inflammatory mediators, 3
Information, provision of, 84, 86–89
   individual requirements, 88–89
Informed consent, 84–85
   form, 97
Infraclavicular approach, percutaneous tunnelled CVC, 116–129
Infusion pumps, 7
   HPN patients, 211, 213–214
   portable, 56, 213
   problems with, 197

Infusion, rate of, 198–199
Infusion time, HPN patients, 217
Innominate vein, hyperosmolar PN solution, 164
Insensible losses, 143, 176
Insertion of catheters
   catheter over the guidewire, 112, 113
   catheter over the guidewire, with or without vein dilator and splittable sheath, 111–112
   catheter over the needle, 110
   catheter through a cannula, 110–111
   catheter through the needle, 109
   and infection rates, 188
   percutaneous, infraclavicular approach, 119–123
Inspecting veins, 8
Insulin
   increase in secretion, 11, 203
   requirements in pancreatitis, 42
   sliding-scale, 178, 182
Intensive care patients, 7, 182, 183, 184
   see also Ventilated patients
Interlink, 162
Internal jugular vein, 61–62, 114
Intestinal failure, 1, 3
   permanent, 15
Intestine, functions, 1, 6
Intralipid, 50
Intravenous hyperalimentation (IVH), 2
Introducing patient to PN, 138, 139
Iodine/iodophors, 159
Isoleucine, 6

J

Jejunostomy, 2
   high-output, 5
   pancreatitis, 41, 42
Jugular veins, 61–62, 92
   catheter misplacement, 126
   catheter over the guidewire technique, with or without vein dilator and splittable sheath, 111–112

K

Kings Fund Report, 39
Kink in catheter, 166, 169, 191, 194
Knowledge of patient, 85
Krebs cycle, 201

L

Laboratory measurements, 9–10
   baseline, 9

Laboratory measurements (*contd*)
HPN patients, 217
patients on PN, 146–147
prior to CVC insertion, 103
Language, 85
Large bowel, assessment of function, 35–36
'Leaky gut', 173
Learning Goals, BAPEN booklet, 207
Length of catheter, 71
measuring patient, 74
Leucine, 6
Lighting, 107
checking, 97
Lignocaine, 118
Link nurse system, 20
Lipaemia, 9
Lipid deposits, 166, 193, 194
removal, 170
Lipids
administration, high liver enzymes, 181
clearance, **148–149**, 180
emulsions, 4, 8, 13, 50
stability, 6–7
maximum infusion rate, 180
metabolism complications, 200–201
side-effects of infusions, **149**
Lipogenesis, 180
Liver
fatty infiltration, 14, 180, 202
high enzymes, manipulation in response,
180–181
liver failure, 175
liver function tests, 10, **149**, 150, 151, 202
Living with PN, patient's perspective,
219–226
case study, 223–225
chronic ill health, 219–222
HPN as long-term therapy, 222
Local anaesthetic
administration for percutaneous CVC
insertion, 118
cream, 91
Long-chain triglycerides (LCT), 181
Long-term parenteral nutrition, 56
hepatobiliary disease, 14
indications, 3
micronutrient deficiencies, 11
monitoring, 9
patient considerations, 57–58
Port-a-Cath insertion, case study, 74–77
see also Home parenteral nutrition
(HPN)
'Loss of self', 225

M

Magnesium, 5, 10, 11, 200
Maintenance of patient on PN, 231–232

Malignancy *see* Cancer
Malnutrition, 32, 139, 227, 228
Material, catheter, 8, 49, 68–70, 165, 166, 188
Mealtimes, difficulties, 152
HPN patients, 225
Median cubital vein, 60
PICC line positioned, **131**
Mediastinum, bleeding into, 127
Medical Control Agency licence, 24
Medications, 96
drug-induced nutritional deficiencies, 33
Medium-chain triglycerides (MCT), 181
Metabolic assessment, 31–32
Metabolic bone disease, 14, 151, 203
Metabolic complications, 11
reduced, dedicated NST/NSC, 25
Metallic taste, 183
Methicillin-resistant *S. aureus*, 156
Microbiologist/infection nurse, **19**
Micronutrients
deficiencies, AIDS patients, 45
screening, HPN patients, 217
Microvilli, 182
Mid-arm circumference measurements, 10,
34, 145, **146**
Minimal enteral feeding (MEN), 7
Misplaced catheters, 126–127
Mobility, reduction in, 152–153
Monitoring, 9–10, 140–147
clinical observation, 141–146
dietetic, 176–178
laboratory observations, 146–147
post percutaneous CVC insertion, 123–126
role of
dietician, 23
pharmacist, 24
self-monitoring, HPN patients, 212,
216–217
specific disease states
gastrointestinal surgery, 42–43
inflammatory bowel disease, 44
pancreatitis, 42
short bowel syndrome, 40
Motivation, NST/NSC team members, 27
Mottled appearance, neck and ears, 165
Mouth
care of, 152
examination, 34, 35
Mucositis, 35
Multidisciplinary team, 17–28, 227–228
benefits of, 24–26
role of, 18–24
success of, 26–28
Multiple lumen catheters, 70, 162
double-lumen cuffed catheter, **79**
infection rates, 188
Multiple organ failure, 173
Muscle wasting, 3, 34
Muscle weakness, 199

N

Nasogastric feeding, 184
  AIDS patients, 45
Nasojejunal feeding, 2
National support groups, 87, 153, 210
Needle phobia, 91
Neonates, excessive amino acids, 14
Nerve damage, 126, 129
Neurological assessment, CVC insertion,
    105–106
Nitrogen, 4
  assessment of requirement, 175
  balance, 147, 177
  effects of overfeeding, 180
Non-steroidal anti-inflammatory agents
    (NSAIDS), 51
Novel substrates, 6
Nursing management, 137–170
  assessment of patient, 139–140
  body image issues, 153
  catheter management guidelines,
      154–170
    catheter damage, 170
    catheter occlusion, 165–170
    detection, prevention and treatment of
        thrombosis, 164–165
    infection, 155–164
    peripheral parenteral nutrition (PPN),
        50–51
  complications associated with PN,
      147–151
    long-term, 150–151
    short-term, 147–150
  cyclical feeding, 7, 8, 151–152
  introducing patient to PN, 138, 139
  learning outcomes for care, 138
  monitoring patient on PN, 140–147
  reduction in mobility, 152–153
  restricted enteral intake, 152
  sleep disturbance, 153–154
  transition to enteral feeding and oral diet,
      154
Nutrient solutions, 4–7
  compounding, 6–7
  delivery, 7–8
  standardised preparations, 26
  see also PN bags
Nutrition
  assessment, 31–35, 39, 51, 106
  calculation of requirements, 140
  complications, 11, 178–181
  monitoring, 10
  see also Dietetic aspects
Nutrition Support Committee (NSC), 17,
    137, 228
Nutrition Support Team (NST), 10, 12, 14,
    17, 39, 137, 228, 232

benefits of, 24–26, 228, 232–233
collective roles, 19
communication, 27
direction of team, 26–27
formal evidence of team's success, 28
individual roles, 19–24
members, 18
motivation of members, 27
observations made by, **19**
referral to, 24

O

Observation of procedure, 98
Occlusion, catheter, 13, 50, 51, 165–170,
    191–195
  causes, 165–166
  detection/diagnosis, 169, 191–193
  nursing care to reduce incidence, 167, **168**
  prevention, 166–167, 193
  treatment, 169–170, 193–194
Occupational therapist, 88
Oedema, 5, 34
  ankle, 217
  pulmonary, 56–57
Operating venue, preparation, 107–109
Operator expertise, CVC insertion, 63–64,
    115, 127, 231
Oral feeding, 7
  pain caused by, diseased pancreas, 41
Osmolality of infusate, 49, 50
Osteoporosis, children, 201
Overfeeding, 179–180
Oxygen therapy, 123

P

Pain
  abdominal, 150
  pancreatitis, 41, 42
  post procedural, 124, 125–126, 141, 196
Pancreatitis, 41–42
Paralytic ileus, burns patients, 46
Particulate matter
  PN bag contamination, 163
  removal, 7, 50
Patient examination, percutaneous CVC
    insertion, 117
Patient's Charter, 84
Patients with existing CVC, 86–87
Patients on Intravenous and Nasogastric
    Nutrition Therapy (PINNT), 153, 210
Percutaneous, tunnelled CVC insertion,
    infraclavicular approach, 116–129
  advantages and disadvantages, 117
  complications, 126–129
  insertion, 119–123

Percutaneous, tunnelled CVC insertion, infraclavicular approach (*contd*)
  creation of subcutaneous tunnel, 120–121
  introducing catheter to vascular system, 121–122
  suturing exit and clavicular sites, 122–123
  postprocedural observations, 123–126
  preparation, 117–119
Peripheral parenteral nutrition (PPN), 7–8, 47–51, 52, 229
  definition 2
Peripheral vein thrombophlebitis (PVT), 8, 48, 52
  prevention, 49–51
Peripheral venous access, 95–96, 107
  veins of arm, 60–61
Peripherally inserted central catheters, (PICC), 56, 59, 212
  definition, 2
  insertion, 65, 66-67, 130, 131–132, 230
    case study, 71–73, 74
    essential requirements, 134
    patient examination, 129–130
    patient preparation, 130
    post procedural observations and complications, 132–133
  length, 71
  lumen size, 70
Personal disruption, illness demands, 224
Personnel role, clinical nurse specialist, 21
Pets, HPN patients, 215
pH of infusate, 49, 50
Pharmacist, **19**, 23–24
  PN bag preparation, 163
Phenytoin, 199
Phlebitis, 67, 133, 163
  see also Peripheral vein thrombophlebitis (PVT)
Phlebotomy, clinical nurse specialist, 21
Phosphate, 5, 10, 11
Photographs, 87
Physical aspects, catheter insertion, 92–93
Physical disfigurement, 225
Plastic carpet protector, 215
Platelet transfusion, 195
PN bags
  48 hour bag, 183
  contamination, 188
  preparation and storage, 163
  split or damaged, 197–198
  standard, 175, 176, 179, 180, 184
Pneumothorax, 124, 126, 127–128, 142, 195–196
Polyethylene catheters, **69**
Polyurethane catheters, 8, 49
  advantages and disadvantages, **69**
Polyvinylchloride (PVC) catheters, 49, 165

advantages and disadvantages, **69**
Port-a-Cath insertion, case study, 74–77
Portable drip stands/infusion pumps, 56, 153, 213
Postpyloric feeding, 47
Potassium, 5
  blood levels, 199
Povidone-iodine, 190
Power points, home assessment, 215
Practising administration, HPN patients, 210–211
Pregnancy, diseases in, 47
Preoperative antibiotics, 96
Preparation *see* Central venous catheters (CVC): preparation for insertion
Pressure dressings, 127, 195
Priming catheter, 120
Prothrombin time, 103
Protocols of care
  CNS responsibility, 20
  sepsis prevention, 189, 190
Proximal veins of arm, 61
Psychological aspects, 93–94
  history taking, 33
  home parenteral nutrition (HPN), 205–207
Pulmonary oedema, 56–57
Pulse, 9, 142
Pulse oximetry, 97, 124
Puncture, arterial/venous wall, 126, 127
Pyrexia, 12, 189

R

Radiation enteritis, 205
Re-siting catheters/cannulae, 8
Reassurance, 90
Refeeding syndrome, 11, 178–179
Referral for PN, 39
  assessing appropriateness, 173–174
Refrigerator, HPN patients, 214, 215
Regular needles, 76
Relatives, presence at insertion, 90
Renal failure, 175
Repairs, catheter, 68, 170, 195
Repeated cannulation, 58
Research
  benefits of NST/NSC expertise, 26
  CNS role, **22**
Resident flora, 158
Resources for PN, 14, 28
Respiratory depression, 91, 123, 124
Respiratory function
  assessment, 104–105
  monitoring, 10, 123–124, 141
Responsibility for care-taking, 221
Retention, sodium and water, 5, 143
Reversing sedation, 91, 123, 124
Rigors, 12

S

Scales, 33
Scars, 93, 225
The Scope of Professional Practice, UKCC, 137–138, 231
Seat belts, 93
Sedation, 91, 106, 107, 123
  administration, percutaneous CVC insertion, 119
Seldinger wire, 65, 111, 112, 120, 121
  arrhythmias caused by, 123
Selection of patients for PN, 37–38, 139, 228
Selenium, 11
Self-care, 93
Self-esteem and physical dependency, 220
Septic patients, 46, 103
  see also Infection, catheter-related
Sexual relations, HPN patients, 93, 206, 212
Sexuality, discussing, 94
Short bowel syndrome, 15, 40–41, 174, 181, 205
  preparation for PN, case study, 99
  weaning from PN, 184
Short-term parenteral nutrition, 56
  case study, PICC insertion, 71–73, 74
  indications, 3
  short-term peripheral feeds, 174
Shoulder tip pain, 124, 125–126, 141, 196
'Sick role' behaviour, 222
Silicone catheters, 75, 165
  advantages and disadvantages, **69**
Single-lumen catheters, 70, 162
  Groshong single-lumen PICC, **66**
Site
  choice of, 92–93
    peripheral parenteral nutrition, 50
  preparation, 95
Size
  of catheters, 70, 165
  of veins, peripheral parenteral nutrition, 50, 67
Skin
  defatting, 160, 190
  observation, 34, 126
Skinfold thickness, 34, 140, 145
Sleep disturbance, 152, 153–154
  HPN patients, 223
Sleeping position, catheter considerations, 57
Small bowel
  assessment of function, 35
  obstruction, PICC case study, 71–73, 74
  resection, 40
Smell of PN, 183
Soap and water, 158
Social aspects, 94–95
  history taking, 33
  role modification

chronically ill person, 220
  HPN patients, 224
Social handwash, 158
Social worker, 88
Society's perception, illness behaviour, 222
Sodium, 5
  depletion, 177
  retention, 143
Sodium chloride flush, 166, 167, 169, 193
Space requirements, CVC insertion, 108–109
Staphylococcus aureus infections, 12, 156, 158, 217
Staphylococcus epidermis infections, 156, 217
Starvation, 3
Steatosis, 14, 180, 202
Steroids
  effect on healing, 123
  glyconeogenesis, 199
Stigma, chronic ill health, 225
Stoma outputs, 175, 177, 184
Stomach, assessment of function, 35
Storage, PN bags, 163
  HPN patients, 212, 214
Strength, 34
  measuring, 144–145
Streptokinase, 13, 165, 193, 194
Subclavian artery, puncture, 127
Subclavian vein, 61, 75, 92
  catheter over the guidewire technique, with or without vein dilator and splittable sheath, 111–112
  repeated access to, 58
Subcutaneous pocket, 75, **76**, 94–95
Subcutaneous port, 59, **76**, 212
  damage to, 13
Subcutaneous tunnel, 59, 63, 112
  case study, silicone CVC insertion, 78–80
  creation of, 120–121, 127
  infection, 156, 189
Sunlight, protecting solutions from, 6, 7
Superior vena cava thrombosis, 165
Supplemental parenteral nutrition (SPN), 2
Supraventricular tachycarida, 124
Surgical placement of CVC, 65–66
Sutures, 122–123, 132, 161, 162
Swimming 79, 94–95
Systemic catheter-related sepsis, 156

T

Tachycardia, 124, 197
Tachypnoea, 147
Taste sensations, 183
Teeth, examination, 34
Teflon catheters, **69**, 70
Temperature, 199
  dysfunction of regulation, 35, 224
  monitoring, 9, 142, 189

Terminology, 85
Thiamin
    administration, 179
    deficiency, 11
Third space losses, 143
Thrombophlebitis *see* Peripheral vein
        thrombophlebitis (PVT)
Thrombosis, 70, 105, 156
    cerebral, 126
    see also Central venous thrombosis (CVT)
Tingling fingers, 126, 129
Tissue plasminogen activator (tPA), 165
Tongue, examination, 34
Topical antibiotics, 160
Total parenteral nutrition (TPN), definition,
        2
Trace elements, 4, 5, 11
    abnormalities, 150, 201–202
    analysis, HPN patients, 217
    monitoring, 178
Training programme, HPN patients,
        210–212
Transient flora, 158
Transmission of microorganisms, 155
Transparent dressings, 51, 160, 161, 190–191
Trauma patients, 47
Trendelenburg position, 98, 105, 106, 118
    patient considerations, 57
Triglycerides
    high serum levels, 200
    medium/long-chain (MCT/LCT), 181
    monitoring, 180
    pancreatitis, 42
Trolleys
    CVC insertion, **108**
    HPN patients, 213

U

Ulcerative colitis, 35, 43
Ultrafine catheters, 49
Urea, 9, 146, 177, 180
Urine
    24 hour collection, 35, 147, 177
        pancreatitis, 42
    analysis, 146, 147, 178, 198
    glycosuria, 198
    output, 143
Urokinase, 12, 13, 165, 169–170, 193, 194

V

Valine, 6

Vancomycin-resistant enterococci, 156
Veins
    availability of suitable, 58–63, 92, 114,
        229
        femoral vein, 62–63
        insertion sites, **59**
        internal jugular vein, 61–62
        jugular veins, 61–62
        peripheral veins of arm, 60–61
        proximal veins of arm, 61
        subclavian vein, 61
        vascular assessment, 105
    daily inspection, 8
    endothelial damage, 164
    size, peripheral parenteral nutrition, 50,
        67
    vascular complications/catheter
        redirection, 126–127
Ventilated patients, 105
    overfeeding, 179
    see also Intensive care patients
Ventricular ectopics, 124
Videos, 86
'Visibility', chronic illness, 221
Vital signs, monitoring, 141–142
Vitamins, 5–6
    monitoring, 178
        in pancreatitis, 42
    vitamin D, metabolic bone disease,
        203
    vitamin B_{12} injections, 181
    vitamin K, 97
        interaction with warfarin, 13
Vitrimix, 174

W

Ward booklet, 87
Warfarin, low-dose, 13, 96, 194
Water, 5
Weaning patient from PN, 181–184, 185
Weighing patients, 33–34, 176
    daily weight, 9, 144
        fluctuations, 176–177
Weight loss, 10, 33, 44
    morbidity, 32
Wernicke's encephalopathy, 179
Withdrawing nutrition, 45
Written information, 86, 87

Z

Zinc deficiency, 201